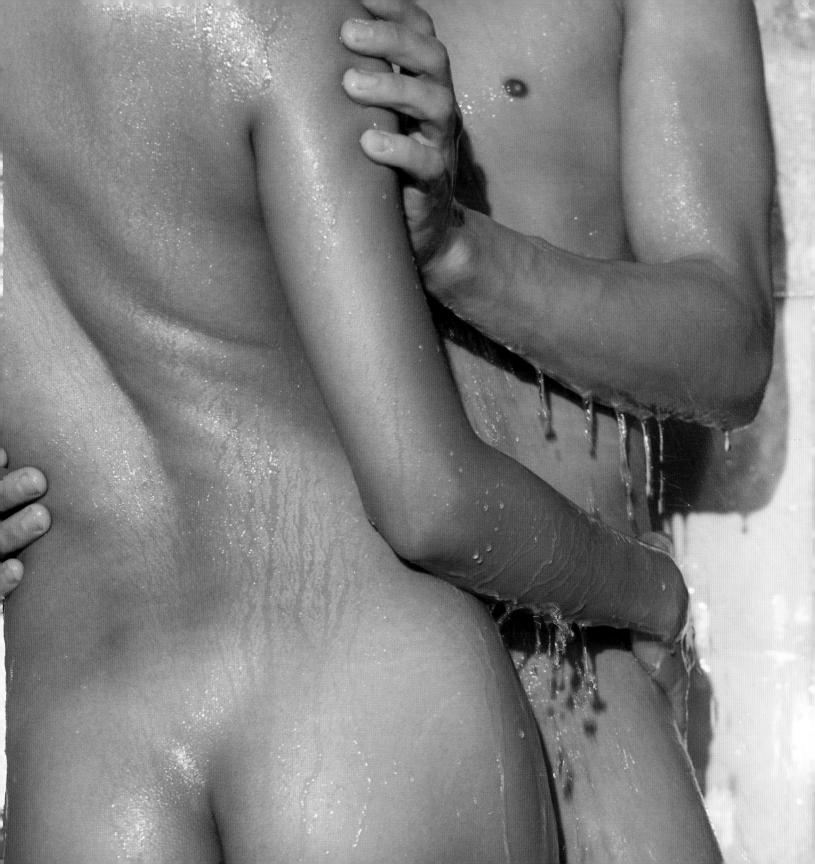

THE NEW
SEX
BIBLE

The Complete Guide to Sexual Love

A QUIVER BOOK

JESSICA O'REILLY, PH.D.

© 2014 Quiver
Photography © 2006, 2014 Quiver

First published in the USA in 2014 by
Quiver, a member of
Quarto Publishing Group USA Inc
100 Cummings Center
Suite 406-L
Beverly, MA 01915-6101
www.quiverbooks.com

The Publisher maintains the records relating to
images in this book required by 18 USC 2257.
Records are located at Rockport Publishers, Inc.,
100 Cummings Center, Suite 406-L, Beverly,
MA 01915-6101.

18 17 16 15 14   2 3 4 5

ISBN: 978-1-59233-603-6

Digital edition published in 2014
eISBN: 978-1-62788-044-2

Library of Congress Cataloging-in-Publication
Data available

Cover design by Burge Agency
Book design by Burge Agency
Photography by Ed Fox, edfox.com, and
Allan Penn

Printed and bound in Hong Kong

Dedication

TO BRANDON.
YOU ROCK.

Contents

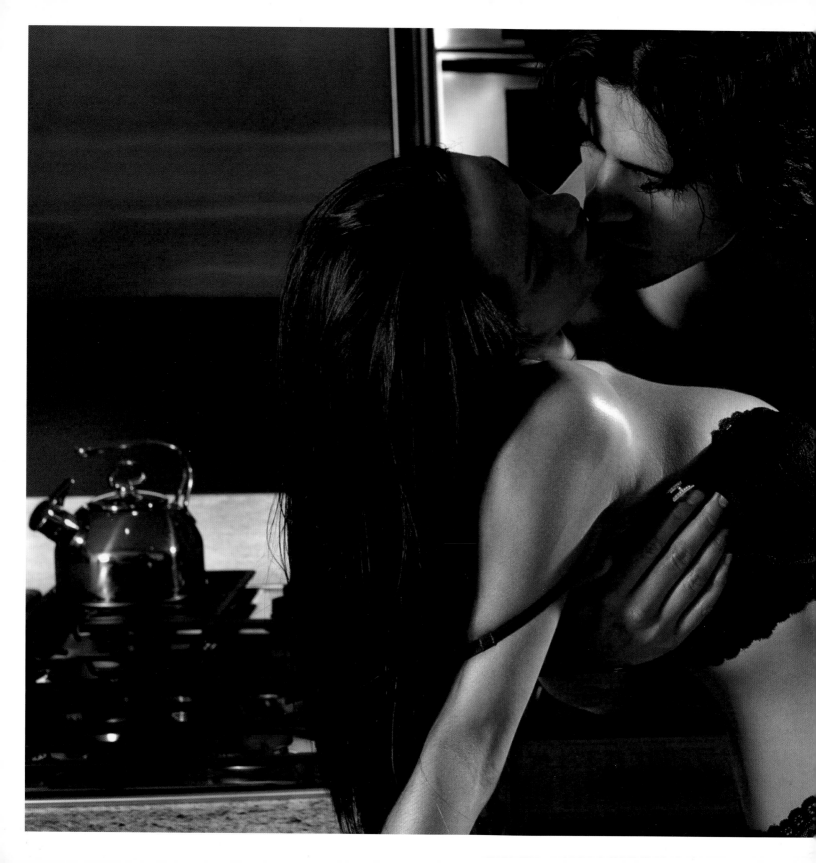

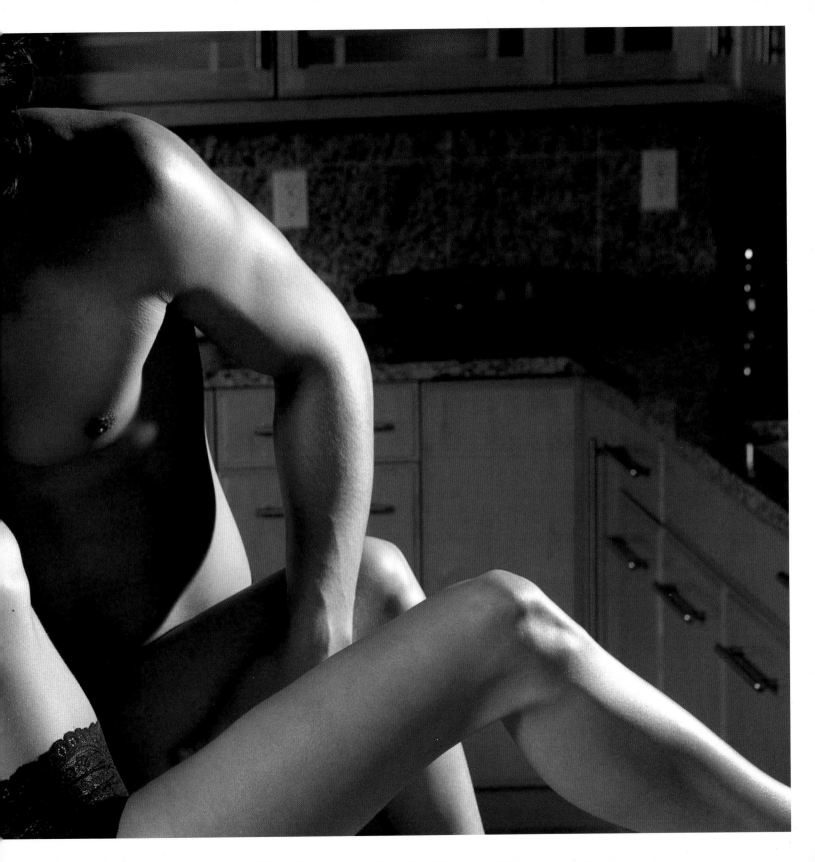

Introduction: About This Book

Welcome to *The New Sex Bible,* your in-depth lovers' guide to all things sexual. Balancing science and anecdote with theory and sure-fire techniques, this handbook is designed to leave you with the knowledge to impress your friends and the skills to astonish your lover. From the latest research findings on orgasm and brain activity during sex to advanced approaches designed for full-body pleasure, I've got you covered.

Chapter 1 covers the scientific basis for the techniques outlined in successive chapters. Though we have a great deal to learn about human sexuality, a new wave of innovative sex researchers armed with MRI technology have led to some groundbreaking discoveries with regard to anatomy, endocrinology, and functioning. And though calculating dopamine levels and uterine angles may not be at the forefront of your thoughts in the bedroom, these foundational findings underpin the seduction, touch, and oral techniques outlined in Chapters 2–3. From learning to flirt and keeping your lover guessing to mastering the Spider Pull massage move and the Twist and Shout blow-job trick, you can rest assured that these techniques are grounded in both science and real-life testing.

Chapter 4 moves on to reveal creative positions to spice up your repertoire, followed by an in-depth chapter exploring the great world of orgasms. Have you ever had a dry orgasm or a spontaneous orgasm? How about an orgasm from fantasy alone? And is faking it ever advisable? The experience of orgasm is complex, personal, and highly varied, and Chapter 5 examines its many permutations.

Moving on to more taboo topics, Chapter 6 unveils novel techniques for anal play, followed by Chapter 7's exploration of toys from tame to kinky. Finally, I share expert advice for overcoming the most common sexual challenges in Chapter 8 and offer practical tools to set you on the path to a lifetime of hot sex in the final pages.

Throughout, you'll also find key information highlighted in various sexpert boxes, which include answers to frequently asked questions, sex tips from the pros, real-life stories, facts for sex geeks, and expert advice based on my experience working with clients both one-and-one and in large group settings.

A note on gender: Throughout *The New Sex Bible*, I alternate between male and female pronouns to describe instructional techniques and scenarios. Because sex and gender roles are fluid, these references are intended as examples only. You can choose to play a variety of roles and switch them up as you see fit, regardless of gender.

From educational programs with special-needs youth to rowdy poolside parties with swingers, I owe the bulk of my expertise and perspective to my clients, who courageously share their most intimate stories, concerns, and revelations. It is from their diverse amalgam of experiences that I draw much of the information contained herein, and I am grateful for their willingness to include me in their process of sexual discovery. Each of our sexual journeys is complex and highly personal, and I am humbled by the fact that you have selected *The New Sex Bible* to be a part of yours.

Read, explore, and practice with pleasure.

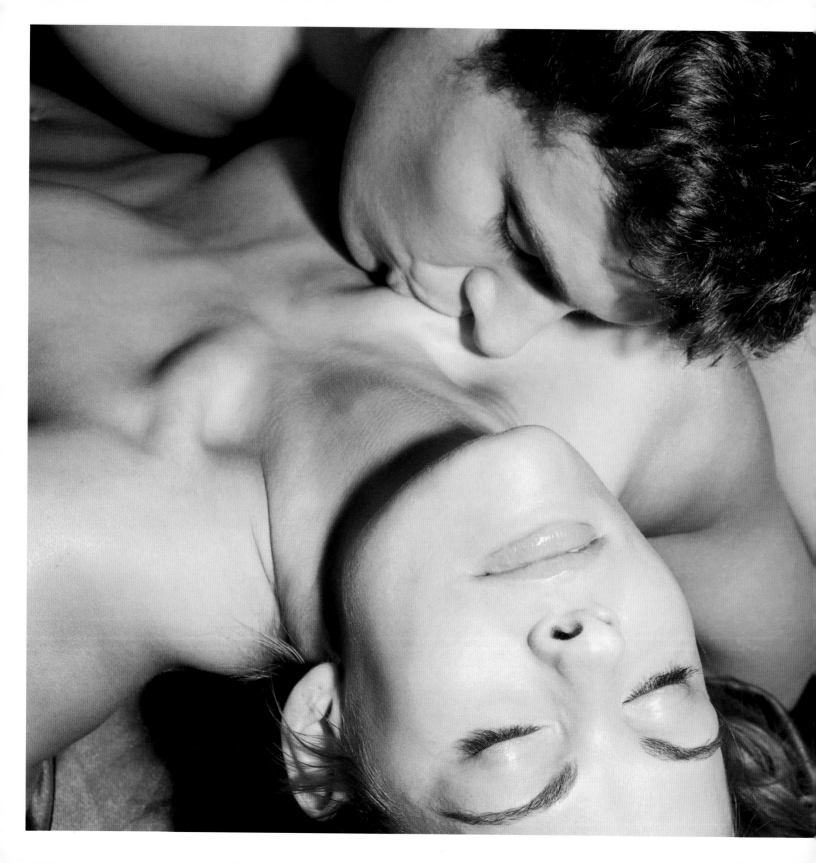

☿ 01 *The Science of Sex*

Sex is an integral component of our social interactions, relationships, and spiritual identities. It shapes the political landscape, informs legislation, and even inspires creative innovation. And, of course, it feels good, too. An intensely physical and undeniably emotional experience, some people consider sex to be the ultimate indulgence of mind and body and the most powerful of human drives. However, despite its central role in our day-to-day lives and our ongoing engagement in sexual activities, many of us know little about the science behind the multitude of sexual experiences in which we partake.

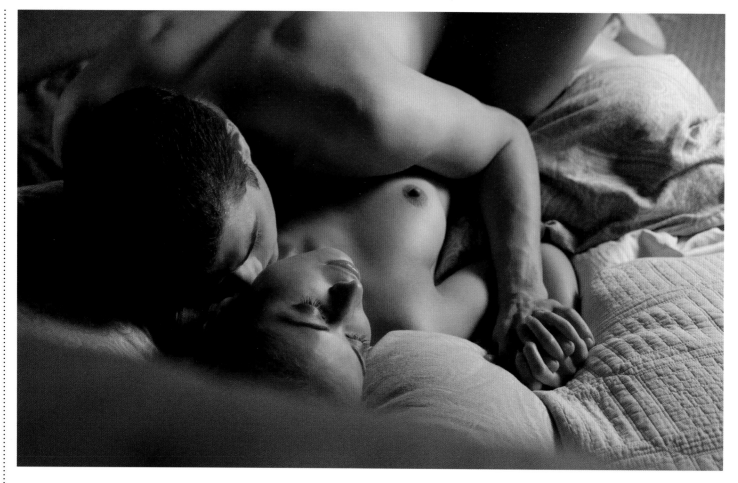

WHY SCIENCE MATTERS TO SEX

In the heat of passion, you probably don't think about why you get an erection or how an orgasm impacts your brain patterns. However, understanding the science of sex can be useful to help you create new sexual scenarios, fine-tune novel techniques, and cultivate sexual relationships that stand the test of time. Science may also offer insight and reassurance when things don't go exactly as planned, as well as help you to generate effective strategies for overcoming common sexual hurdles. For example, some basic understanding of the clitoris's full anatomy might shed some light on why most women don't orgasm during intercourse and help you to discover positions that stimulate the sensitive clitoral bulbs. And as you learn more about the role of contractions in orgasm and ejaculation, you may develop a better understanding of how to intensify pleasure through simple pulse sensations.

You obviously don't want to flood your mind with thoughts of hormones, chemicals, and physiological processes *while* you're having sex, but as your knowledge of sexual science increases, so too will your sexual self-esteem. This confidence boost will not only broaden your horizons but also inspire you to explore sex and experience pleasure in new and exciting ways.

YOUR BRAIN ON SEX

The pituitary gland lights up. The nucleus accumbens and ventral tegmental areas are activated. The hypothalamus goes into overdrive. And the center of reasoning and behavior shuts down as you spiral into the euphoria of sexual pleasure! All this activity might sound like sensory overload, but this is actually your brain … on sex.

Though the heart is often thought to represent matters of love and sex, this vital organ's involvement in sexual processes is minimal in comparison to that of the brain and the nervous system. PET scans of the brain during sexual activity and orgasm reveal that its reward circuit lights up with a flurry of activity during sex. These scans confirm that sex is both a physical and emotional experience, as the amygdala, which controls emotion, as well as the area that manages muscle function, are activated.

Brain studies also explain why sex is so pleasurable from a chemical perspective, as the areas related to dopamine release become hotbeds for sexual activity, resulting in increased levels of this feel-good neurotransmitter. And as the pituitary gland is activated, the release of endorphins, oxytocin, and vasopressin promote pain reduction, intimacy, and bonding. These observable brain reactions may not help you to perfect your sexual technique, but they might help you to understand your emotions before, during, and after sex.

The power sex wields over our minds and bodies is also evidenced in our brain activity. Sex is so overwhelmingly exciting, pleasurable, and rewarding that our brains during orgasm look almost identical to a brain on heroin. According to neuroscientist Dr. Gert Holstege, there is only a 5 percent difference between our brain's observable reaction to sex and heroin, which may explain the euphoric high we experience after a passionate sex session. And since the lateral orbitofrontal cortex, which is the section behind the left eye responsible for sound decision-making, turns off completely during orgasm, we often toss reason to the wind when the prospect of sex presents itself. Though it may seem risky to allow our animal instincts to take over as we set logic aside in favor of pleasure, a degree of letting go and losing control is essential to desire, arousal, and orgasm.

FOR SEX GEEKS

The *cortical homunculus* is a map of the brain that illustrates which parts of its sensory and motor cortices correspond to various parts of our bodies. It was first developed by Dr. Wilder Penfield, and contemporary researchers postulate that nongenital orgasms may be related to brain layout and the activation of sensory cortical regions. For example, when organs are injured or removed, remapping of the senses may occur, allowing us to experience sexual and orgasmic sensations in other body parts.

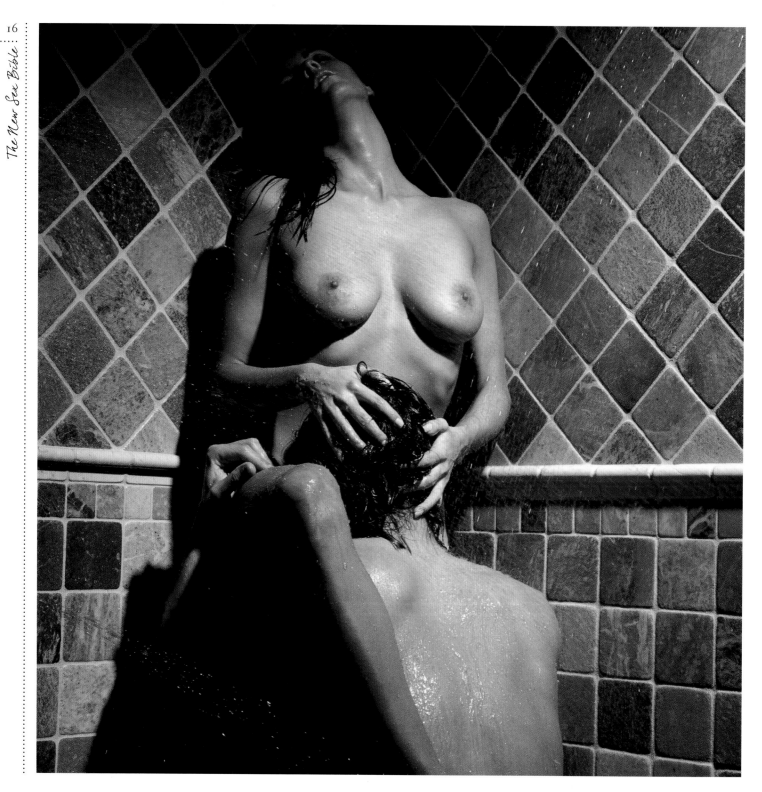

THE ROLE OF NERVES

The brain may be your most powerful sex organ, but nerves are the airwaves that transmit signals so that you can experience pleasure. Though nerve endings throughout your entire body can contribute to sexual sensations and orgasm, the following large nerves communicate information from the genitals to the brain: The pelvic nerve transmits sensations from the vagina and cervix in women and the rectum and bladder in both men and women; the vagus nerve communicates signals from the cervix, uterus, and vagina, bypassing the spinal cord; the pudendal nerve carries information from the clitoris, penis, and scrotum; and the hypogastric nerve transmits data from the uterus, cervix, and prostate. These distinct nerve pathways illustrate the complexity of sexual response and orgasm and support anecdotal evidence of orgasms from various sources of stimulation.

YOUR BODY ON SEX: THE SEXUAL RESPONSE CYCLE

While your brain is awash in an eruption of erotic activity during sex, your body's response is equally complex and remarkable. Early sex researchers William Masters and Virginia Johnson studied sexual response by observing live sex acts and documenting changes in the body. They divided the sexual response cycle into four stages: excitement, plateau, orgasm, and resolution. Sex therapist Helen Singer Kaplan later proposed a three-phase model (desire, excitement, and orgasm), noting that sexual response is also cognitive and psychological. These linear models inspired alternative frameworks including circular cycles that acknowledge the role of seduction, emotional intimacy, and relationship satisfaction in sexual response.

As sexual response undoubtedly involves the interaction of both emotional and physiological processes, I have added the anticipation stage to this updated model. However, the cycle of sexual response is highly varied and the following framework is a general guide. You will find that your unique responses vary from experience to experience, and you don't necessarily have to undergo each stage or physical symptom during every sexual episode.

Anticipation is often the hottest part of sex. When planning a vacation, the preparatory rituals (reading hotel reviews, shopping for resort wear, and scouting the top attractions) can be just as exciting as the vacation itself. The physical changes that occur may not be visible during sexual anticipation, but they are significant nonetheless. Anticipation of reward has been shown to activate several parts of the brain, including the pleasure center, which controls the

DR. JESS SAYS . . .

It's one thing to read that part of the brain shuts down during orgasm and a whole other thing to *experience* it. I recently met a woman who actually wore this experience on her sleeve in the form of a massive self-inflicted bruise. The night before our meeting, she had bit herself so hard during sex that the bruise spread three full inches across. She was so preoccupied by the pleasure that she didn't even notice it until the next morning.

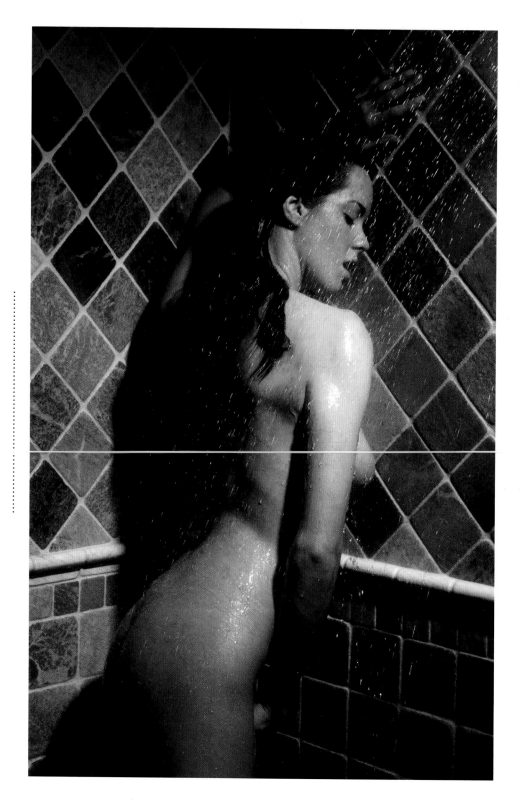

release of dopamine. Scientists also believe that as we anticipate sex in our minds or encounter cues that have previously led to pleasure, our bodies become better-prepared for the physical experience on account of classical conditioning.

Desire often precedes excitement, but we can experience desire in many ways. You may yearn for a gentle touch that culminates in a long cuddling session, or you might crave rough penetration, biting, and spanking. There is no predicting the trajectory of your desires, and their intensity can ebb and flow during the course of sex play. We often assume that sex involves a steady climb toward climax, but this is not always the case. You may experience intense desire that tapers off before plateau, or you may even engage in intimate relations without initially experiencing desire.

During the EXCITEMENT phase of sexual response, your body often undergoes a variety of visible changes. Blood flow to the genitals, breasts, and lips results in swelling and color change in these areas. This increased flow to the surface of the skin produces a sex flush. The vagina begins to lubricate as the clitoris swells and the uterus tents upward. In the man, the penis becomes erect and the testes elevate as the scrotum contracts. The nipples harden and your breath, heart, and blood pressure rates climb.

During the PLATEAU phase, signs of excitement heighten further. The clitoral glans retracts beneath its hood. The outer third of the vagina swells and the uterus continues to tent upward. Muscular tension, heart rate, breathing, and blood pressure continue to increase. The testicles elevate closer to the body, and muscles may begin to spasm.

Considered the climax of sexual activity, the experience of ORGASM varies greatly not only from person to person but also between each sexual episode. Physical reactions might include a sense of pleasurable release as your mind becomes wholly focused on the physical experience. Orgasm is also reached by involuntary muscular contractions throughout

the pelvic region. These contractions are spaced at an average of 0.8 seconds apart, beginning at 0.6 seconds and slowing down thereafter. The pupils dilate in response to oxytocin release into the spinal cord area that controls this response. In the man, expulsion of fluid through the urethra results in ejaculation.

During the RESOLUTION phase, the body begins to return to its unaroused state, and swelled and erect body parts return to their usual size and color. Some people experience fatigue, while others can reengage rapidly with sexual activity. Men often need time to recover, known as the *refractory period*, which varies between men and tends to increase with age.

"I used to be totally grossed out by my nether regions. I didn't like the way they felt or looked, so I did my homework and sat spread eagle in front of a full-length mirror every morning while doing my makeup. I think I became desensitized and within ten days, my 'ick factor' dropped from an 8 to a 4."

—Tara, 22

ALL ABOUT HER

We often refer to a woman's genitals as her vagina, but for many women it is the vulva from which they derive the greatest experience of pleasure. Thanks to a culture that shrouds sex in secrecy, some people have never heard of the vulva, and others assume that vagina and vulva are one and the same. This is a shame, as getting to know your body (and your lover's) increases the likelihood of desire, arousal, and orgasm.

VULVA VERSUS VAGINA

The *vagina* is the stretchable, tube-like canal on the *inside* that connects the uterus (via the cervix) to the outside world. It is a muscular structure that is more accurately described as a potential space than an open hole. Some people compare it to an uninflated balloon, as in a relaxed state, its walls generally touch and during arousal it becomes larger to make space for objects of pleasure. Composed of expandable tissue, it functions as a protective barrier, a passageway for birth, and a penetrable organ of pleasure during sexual activity.

The *vulva* refers to all of the delicious parts on the *outside* including the outer lips, inner lips, clitoral glans/head, clitoral hood, vestibule, urethral opening, vaginal opening, and mons/pubic mound. Because of its relationship to the clitoris (see page 26), this outer region is a potential hotbed of orgasmic activity, and many of the finger and tongue techniques described in Chapter 3 focus on this soft, warm, and supersensitive region.

If you haven't taken a good look at your vulva lately, now is the perfect time to get to know her. Use a hand mirror or sit in front of a full-length mirror and use your fingers to locate your outer lips, inner lips, clitoris, and pubic mound. You may need two hands to open your inner lips and reveal the shiny vestibule where you'll find the vaginal and urethral openings. It is not uncommon for a woman to have trouble visually locating her clitoris, as it is not a body part that most of us learn about from a young age. As you pull up gently on the skin at the top of your inner labia (just below your pubic mound) you will find your sensitive clitoral head. It is usually round and a bit shiny and protrudes from beneath the hood. Every woman's body is different, so yours may poke out conspicuously or only extend slightly from beneath its hood.

Your vulva is a part of your sexual fingerprint and thus no two are alike. Your lips will vary from every other woman's in color, thickness, shape and length, as will the hood of your clitoris. Some women report dissatisfaction with the appearance of their vulva (and their inner labia in particular), but experts report that repeated self-exams can help increase comfort levels and improve women's relationships with their genitals. If you feel uncomfortable with your vulva, take your time examining it in the mirror and repeat this exercise daily to become better acquainted with its appearance and function.

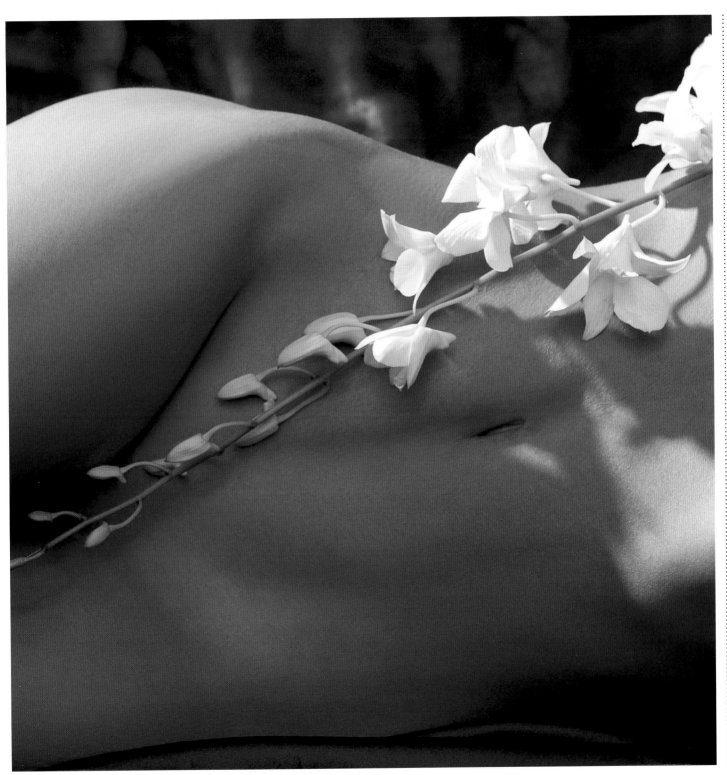

REAL PEOPLE, REAL SEX

"People ask me why I have lasered off all of my pubic hair. I mean, I'm a middle-aged mom, not a porn star anywhere other than my own mind. But something magical happened for me when I did. It was the first time that I really saw my labia in all their glory. And the feeling was incredible. I tell people that it's the difference between having someone kiss me on the top of my head and having someone kiss me on my lips. Honestly, it was the most fully connected to my sexual self that I ever felt, and I never wanted it hidden again." —Alyssa Royse, host of Sexxx Talk Radio

A TOUR OF THE VULVA

The *outer labia* border the left and right sides of the vulva and span from just above the perineum to the pubic bone. They may be covered in hair and contain sensitive nerve endings and erectile tissue. Just above the top of where the outer lips meet, you'll find the *mons* or pubic mound, which is an area of fatty skin where pubic hair grows. Just below, you'll see the *clitoral hood*, which protects the highly sensitive *clitoral glans/head* and is connected to the *shaft* by a small notch of skin called the *frenulum*.

The *inner labia* are hairless, thin lips that protect the vulval vestibule, vaginal opening, and *urethral meatus* (pronounced *mee-ay-tus*). They come in many shapes, lengths, and colors, and it is normal for them to be two different sizes. The *fourchette* is the point at which the inner labia meet at the southernmost point.

If you open the inner lips, you'll reveal the *vulval vestibule*, which is shiny and outlined around the edges by *hart's line*. It is the site of the *urethral meatus*, which is the hole through which women pee and ejaculate. The *vaginal opening* is also located within the vulval vestibule just below the urethra and most of the sensitive nerve endings are located near this opening. The *U-spot* is also located in the vulval vestibule in an upside-down U position surrounding the urethra.

The *Bartholin's glands* are two small secretion glands near the bottom of the vulva, with ducts on either side of the vaginal opening. They are located under the skin, and they produce a very small amount of fluid to lubricate the vulva.

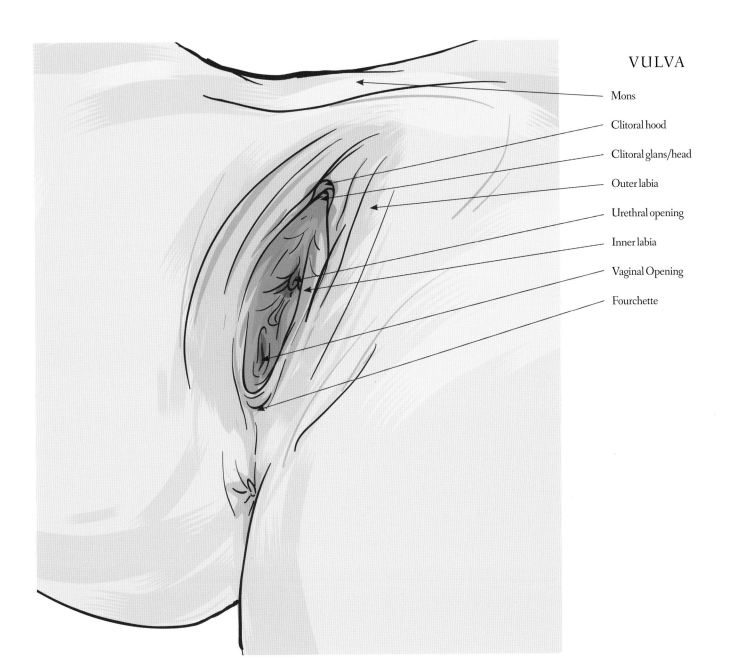

VULVA

Mons

Clitoral hood

Clitoral glans/head

Outer labia

Urethral opening

Inner labia

Vaginal Opening

Fourchette

SEX TIPS FROM THE PROS

Kegel exercises involve the contraction and release of your pelvic floor muscles, and the potential benefits are many: greater continence, improved circulation to the pelvic region, greater orgasmic control (and the possibility of multiples), stronger ejaculations, and more powerful orgasms. To contract your pelvic floor muscles and perform a Kegel, picture yourself pulling your genitals upward. Women can think about sucking air into the vagina or they can insert a finger and clench the muscles around it to contract. Men can envision pulling their testicles upward or lifting the penis slightly to tense these muscles. You will even see the penis rise slightly as you contract, which will be more visible with an erection.

If you have difficulty finding the right muscles, you can try stopping the flow of urine while peeing to identify the sensation of contraction. However, for health reasons, you don't want to repeatedly interrupt urination, so use this approach as a one-time learning tool. Because Kegels involve the contraction of the pelvic floor, it is important to emphasize the release/relaxation equally. Some experts suggest traditional squat exercises are equally important to improving pelvic floor health and alignment. Kegel exercises do not offer a one-size-fits-all approach to muscle health, so if you have the opportunity to see a pelvic floor therapist, please do! They have the expertise to help identify the best pattern of exercises for your specific needs.

INSIDE THE VAGINA

Just because you can't see these highly sensitive regions doesn't mean you shouldn't explore them, either on your own or with your honey.

G-Spot

This sensitive area along the upper wall of the vagina (toward the stomach) has enjoyed its share of controversy over the years. Dr. Beverly Whipple named the G-spot after Ernst Grafenberg, MD, who previously described it as a "distinct erotogenic zone." The G-spot is an area marked by many sensitive nerve pathways, tissues, and organs, but it is not a distinct entity, nor is it located *inside* of the vagina. Dr. Whipple clarifies that it can be felt *through* the vagina and, when stimulated, the tissue begins to swell. As opposed to being a singular organ, it is believed that its sensitivity is connected to corollary stimulation of the female prostate (composed of glands associated with female ejaculation), urethral sponge (erectile tissue that surrounds the urethra), and inner clitoris.

A-Spot

Beyond the G-spot in the vaulted space between the front wall of the vagina and cervix, you'll find the anterior fornix erogenous zone, also known as the A-spot. According to Malaysian researcher Dr. Chua Chee Ann, stimulation of the A-spot can result in increased lubrication and sexual pleasure. He suggests inserting a clean, lubricated finger or toy into the vagina along the upper wall and reaching to the deepest point.

While you're in there, you can also move your fingers around to locate your cervix, which may feel round, rubbery, and a bit firmer than the rest of the vagina.

Cul-de-Sac

Located opposite the A-spot on the back wall of the vagina at its deepest point, this sensitive region is associated with dual stimulation of the vagina and the rectum. As the uterus tents upward during sexual response, the cul-de-sac may become more responsive to pressure and stimulation.

Cervix

Connecting the vagina and the uterus is the small cylinder-shaped cervix that plays a role in both reproductive function and sexual pleasure. Though some women find direct pressure on their cervix uncomfortable, others respond with orgasmic pleasure to deep touch. It is not uncommon for a woman's experience of pleasure to fluctuate with her menstrual cycle, and many report that stimulating the cervix with a penis or toy is more pleasurable if her arousal levels are already heightened.

Pelvic Floor Muscles

The pelvic floor muscles form a sling to support the lower pelvis and are integral to sexual functioning in both men and women. Composed of three layers of muscle, a well-toned set of pelvic floor muscles promotes continence, flexibility, and greater orgasmic control.

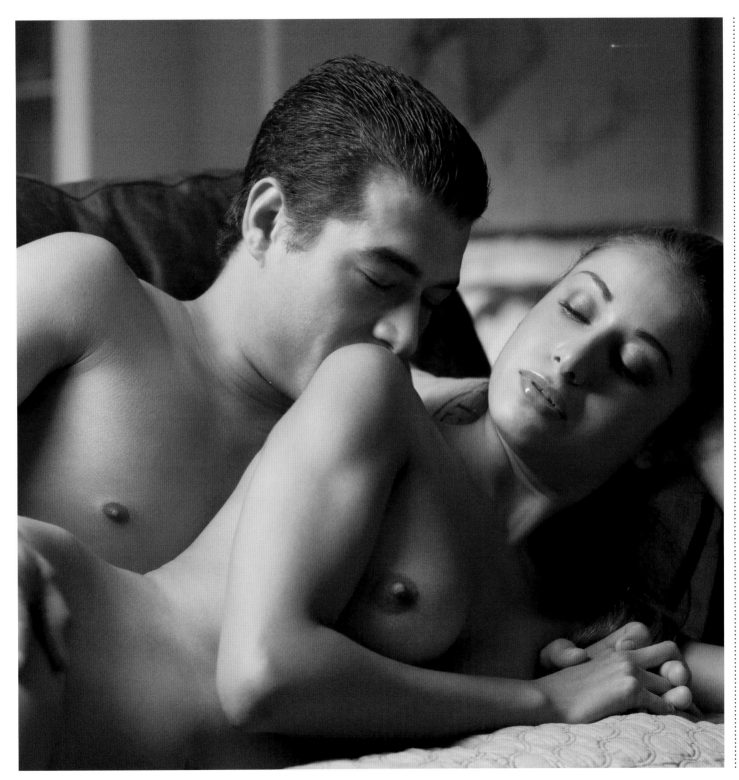

THE CLITORIS EXPOSED

You've probably heard a great deal about the clitoris, and you likely already know that it exists solely for the purpose of pleasure. But did you know that the clitoris has legs? And that the complex structure of the clitoris may explain why most women orgasm from rubbing, grinding, and pressing on the vulva?

The clitoris is more than just a tiny nodule at the top of where the labia meet. That shiny pearl-like structure is actually only the *head* of the clitoris. It also has two legs, two bulbs, foreskin, glans, a shaft, and the capacity to become erect. Once you study the full anatomy of the clitoral complex, you may conclude that the clitoris is much like a penis . . . only smaller. But when you further examine the deep roots and multiple parts of the inner clitoris, it becomes more obvious that the clitoris isn't a smaller version of the penis at all but simply a variant model.

Both the clitoris and the penis are derived from the same tissue in utero. An examination of the clitoris's many parts and their functions reveals further shared attributes between the male and female sex organs.

The *glans* is the head of the clitoris that protrudes from beneath the hood to varying degrees, depending on a woman's unique makeup and her arousal levels. As previously mentioned, we often mistake this pea-sized bump for the entire clitoris and because it can be highly sensitive to touch, it is protected by the clitoral hood (or *foreskin*). The *shaft* is attached to the clitoral glans and composed of erectile tissue that fill with blood just like the penis. That's right: Women get boners, too!

The clitoral *legs* and *bulbs* are part of the inner clitoris, and the legs can extend several inches. They point toward the thighs when relaxed and then stretch backward during arousal, allowing the clitoris to double in size as it becomes engorged with blood. The *bulbs* or *vestibules* of the clitoris underlie the labia and also swell with excitement. As they expand, they cause the vulva to expand outward and create a tight sensation around the outer third of the vagina, which Masters and Johnson named the *orgasmic platform*.

Women often complain that their lovers treat the clitoris like an elevator button. *Press and release. Press and release.* Now that you are familiar with the anatomy of the entire clitoral complex, you likely understand why this approach might be less than thrilling. Poking against the glans of the clitoris is comparable to pressing on the head of the penis: It's not the worst move ever, since someone is touching your dick, but those hands could certainly be put to better use.

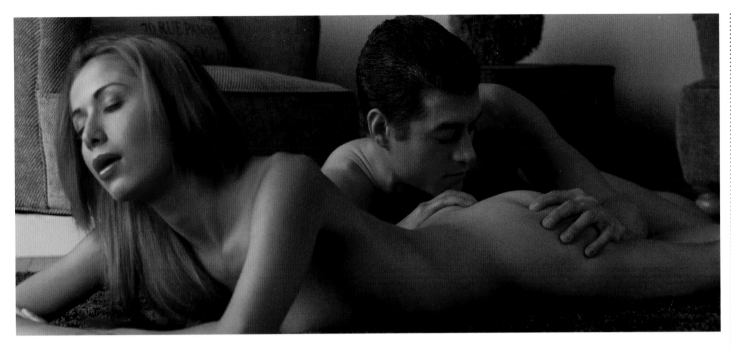

GETTING COMFORTABLE IN YOUR SKIN

The way you feel about your body is intrinsically related to your experience of sexual pleasure. Research continues to confirm that those who feel most comfortable in their skin report the highest levels of sexual functioning, and that negative thoughts about your body can impede orgasm. And since body image is all about how you *feel* about your body as opposed to what your body *looks* like, a hotter body does not amount to a hotter sex life. However, a positive *attitude* toward your body might be just what the sex doctor ordered.

Developing a healthy relationship with your body doesn't mean that you have to idealize every square inch. Positive body image involves seeing your own beauty and learning to see your body as functional—both physically and erotically.

Here are some strategies for improving the way you see your body.

Surround yourself with positive friends, family, and peers. Much like happiness, science suggests that attitudes toward our bodies may be contagious. One study of 150 women found that our own body image and emphasis on weight loss is linked to our perception of how our friends feel about their bodies. So avoid commiserating with friends about a pound or two lost or gained and hang out with people who don't make their appearance a central focus.

Exercise. Physical activity isn't only tied to body image in terms of the impact it can have on your weight, shape, size, and appearance. More important, exercise releases feel-good endorphins, and research suggests that even short-term exercise can change the way you *feel* about your appearance. In one study, both men and women reported feeling fitter, healthier, and more satisfied with their bodies after just six forty-minute workout sessions. This shift in attitude occurred regardless of the fact that neither their weight nor their shape changed over the course of the study.

Develop healthy stress-coping skills. But what does this have to do with sex and body image? According to experts: everything. Developmental psychologist and body image researcher from the University of Arizona, Shannon Snapp, Ph.D., found that those who have constructive skills to manage stress are less likely to develop poor eating or over-exercising habits that can reinforce negative body image.

Masturbate! Self-pleasure and self-esteem are positively correlated, so reach down there and soothe yourself into a frenzy of warm, fuzzy feelings! When your body performs for you, whether through daily tasks, sports, or sexual pleasure, you tend to feel better about its appearance and function.

FAQ: I LIKE TO
MASTURBATE, BUT IT
MAKES MY HUSBAND
JEALOUS. HOW CAN I
TALK TO HIM ABOUT
THIS AND MAKE HIM
UNDERSTAND THAT IT'S
NOTHING TO WORRY
ABOUT?

Ruth Neustifter, Ph.D., a marriage and family therapist (aka Dr. Ruthie), says, "You're facing a very common problem for people of all genders. One of the best ways to handle this kind of jealousy is to have a lighthearted talk where nobody problem solves. Invite him to tell you what is behind the jealousy so you can listen and ask questions without judgment. Getting it off his chest might help quite a bit. It may be that he feels that he should be able to provide for all of your sexual needs and is afraid of failing you. Perhaps he feels that it's wrong for him to masturbate and carries that over to you. Or it may be something else. Once you both understand his concerns it will be easier to address them directly. Masturbation is good for your mind and body, and even better when both of you are happy about it. Remember, though: You have every right to feel good about pleasuring yourself, and you don't need anybody else's permission!"

UNCOVER HER EROGENOUS ZONES

Erogenous zones are hot spots on the body that tend to be highly responsive to sexual touch. In reality, the whole body is a massive, potential erogenous zone, but there are some areas that tend to be especially reactive when stimulated. Her breasts and genitals may be the most obvious areas, but if you take some time to explore the erotic wonderland of her body, you'll discover that you can make her squirm, moan, and beg for more by kissing and caressing her sexy body parts that are often deprived of affection.

As you explore the many regions of her beautiful body, experiment with different strokes, touches, kisses, and breaths, gradually increasing the pressure and tempo as her arousal heightens. Play with the following erogenous zones to see which ones she responds to and revisit them every so often to see how her interpretations of pleasure change over time.

Ears

Not only are her ears sensitive to the sound of your voice and the flick of your tongue, but the anticipation of your kiss can send shivers down her spine. Breathe very gently over the sides of her neck and ears before circling your tongue around the edges.

Collarbone

The clavicle and the shallow grooves above it can be highly responsive to light touch. The small depressions below it are considered acupressure points that trigger relaxation to facilitate sexual response. Run the pads of your fingers over the bone and your tongue along the underside before making your way to her breasts.

Suprasternal Notch

Also known as the jugular notch, this is the triangular dip at the base of her neck centered above her collarbone. It is considered an erogenous zone for both its sensual appearance and hypersensitivity. Since it overlies her airway, you'll want to take caution to kiss her gently as you swivel your tongue around the indentation.

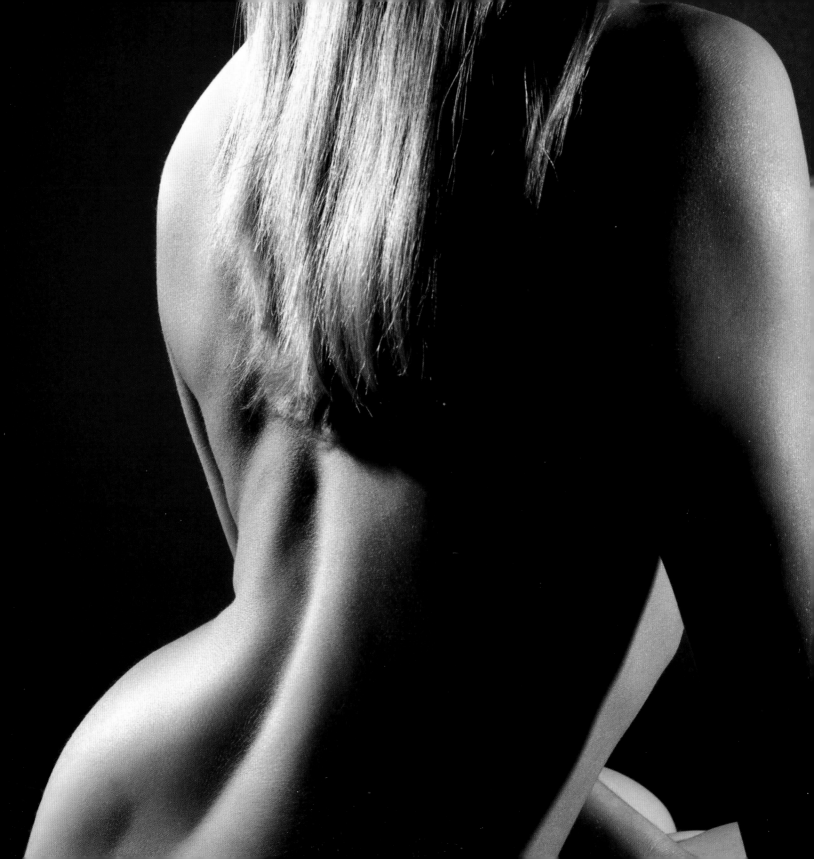

Philtrum

From the Latin for *love potion,* this small groove above the center of her lips has long been considered an erogenous zone. Plant the softest kiss possible on this area before running your tongue along the line of her upper lip, known as cupid's bow.

Lower Back

Some women say that their lower back is the most sensitive area of their body, and a handful report that tickling this area can result in intense arousal and even orgasmic sensations. Sweep your palms in wide circular motions over her lower back to prime her for some playful hip grabbing and primal thrusting.

Crook of Her Elbow

This thin-skinned region is the division between the friend-zone of the upper arm and lover's lane, the lower arm leading down to her fingertips. Slide your finger against it seductively while out for dinner as you look her in the eye or hold her down by her inner elbows while she is screaming with pleasure.

Backs of Her Knees

Make her weak in the knees and tingly in all the right places by awakening this sensitive zone with a featherlight touch. Trace figure-eight patterns over this thin-skinned patch with a silk scarf or small feather while blowing gentle kisses between her thighs from behind.

Ankles

Just below the anklebone on the inside of the foot, you'll find a hollowing that is considered a reflexology point connected to her vagina. While performing cunnilingus, reach down and circle your thumb around this area to activate its sexual reflex.

Eyelids

The area around her eyes likely receives little in the way of sexual attention, but her eyelids and the soft pads beneath her eyes can be highly responsive to gentle touch. With nerves very close to the surface and thin skin without significant subcutaneous fat (similar to that of the scrotum), the eyelids seem to be designed for pleasure. Flutter your lashes teasingly against hers or swipe your fingers gently across her lids to encourage her to relax and take in the sensations of pleasure.

Bellybutton

The positioning of her navel in proximity to her mons, coupled with the density of nerve endings in the region, makes this sensitive indentation a common erogenous zone. Some women say they experience sensations in their clitoris through the bellybutton, which may be attributable to a nerve pathway that connects it to the spine through the pelvic region. Spiral your tongue around its perimeter before sliding it in and sucking gently with your lips against her tummy.

Pucker

The sensitive bum hole (anus) is highly erogenous for many women and men. Rich in nerve endings, it is reactive both to light touch and heavy pressure. (I cover this erotic hot spot in greater depth in Chapter 6.)

REAL PEOPLE, REAL SEX

"My hunt for the clitoris was purposeful. I was always taught to keep my hands away from down there, and, honestly, touching it really grossed me out. When I finally saw the little 'ball' [head] of my clit, I was relieved. I always knew it was there, because I had rubbed it with my dildo plenty of times, but seeing it was kind of reaffirming. There is something about knowing and understanding your own body that puts you at ease." —Tammy, 24

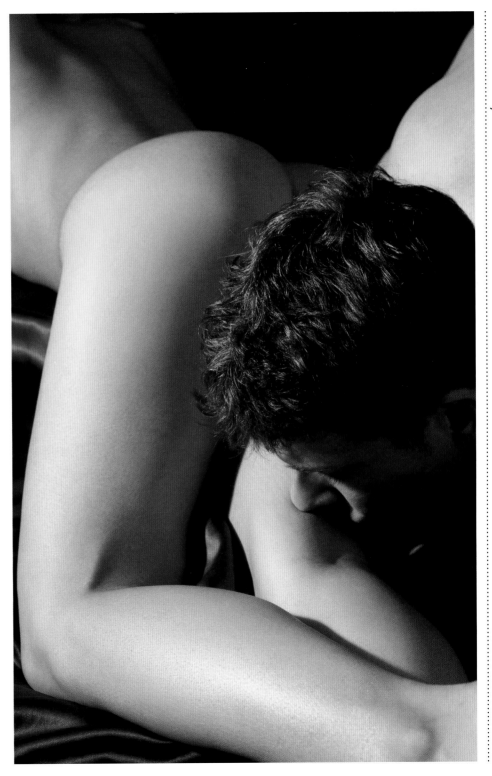

PERSONAL PLEASURE MAP

Every woman's path to personal pleasure is unique and winding, so draw him a map to help guide the way. Use the diagram at right to highlight the areas you experience as erogenous to express both *where* and *how* you enjoy being stimulated.

Taking time to explore your body can help reveal new and sometimes surprising pathways to pleasure. We often assume that the breasts and genitals are our exclusive or primary sources of sexual pleasure, but the reality is that the experience of arousal and orgasm can occur from a range of sources. If you don't have the time or patience to slowly caress your entire body and take note of specific sensations, try breaking each section down into a single session. Consider repeating this exercise periodically to observe the ways in which your body's unique experiences of pleasure change over time.

Color each area according to your preferences:

Yellow indicates you enjoy a soft, gentle caress or kiss of the area.

Blue suggests that you prefer a firm touch or fondle.

Green demarcates the regions where you like a wetter, deeper kiss.

Purple shows the spots that desire ...

(You fill in the blank.)

Red areas are off-limits to all touch.

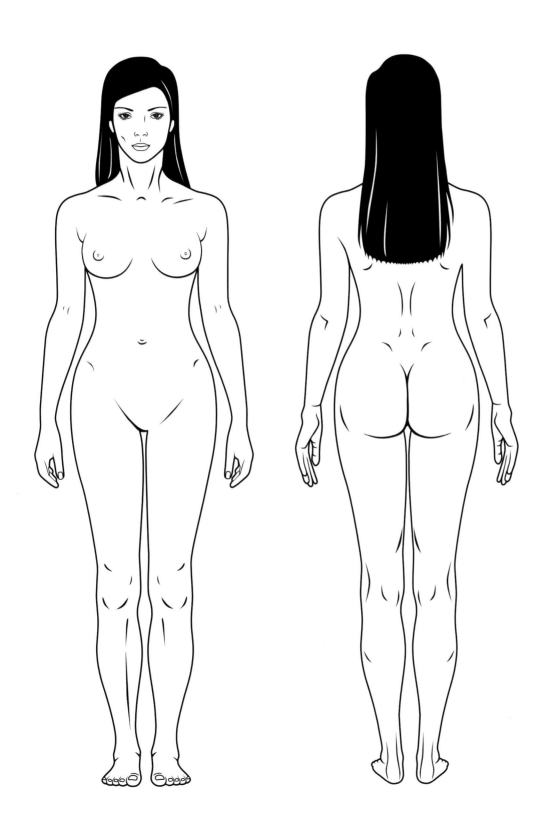

ALL ABOUT HIM

The penis is a central feature of all things sexual and is often revered as a symbol of virility. But male sexuality is not limited to this one region—as wonderful as it may be. Men also derive pleasure from a range of erogenous zones, and full-body orgasms usually require that you pay attention to these oft-neglected pleasure spots.

We often conclude that a hard penis is a sure-fire sign of arousal, but it is possible to get an erection in an unaroused state, and the absence of an erection is not necessarily a sign of disinterest. The body works in mysterious ways and there are many factors that affect erections.

FOR SEX GEEKS

The process of erection involves a complex interplay of the parasympathetic (involuntary) nerves, blood flow, and oxytocin-containing neurons. In response to stimulation, the arteries that lead into the penis open, allowing pressurized blood to enter while the veins that carry blood away from the penis constrict. Blood is trapped in the two corpora cavernosa, causing the shaft to grow and harden. This process is facilitated by impulses along the dorsal nerve, which activate the cavernous nerve.

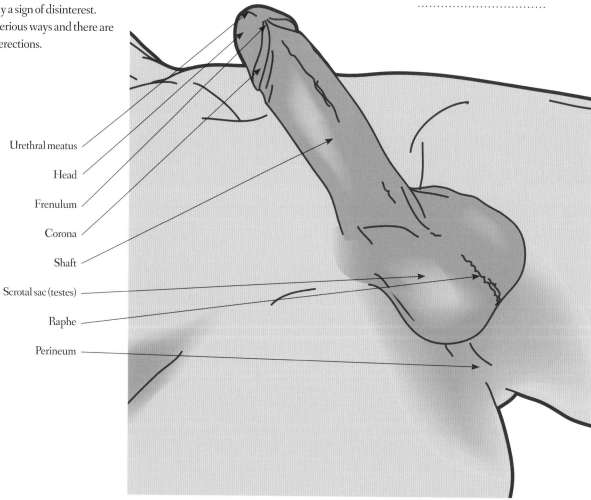

Urethral meatus

Head

Frenulum

Corona

Shaft

Scrotal sac (testes)

Raphe

Perineum

PENIS, PROSTATE, AND BALLS, OH MY!

The penis is a sensitive organ, and it varies greatly from man to man in terms of shape, size, curve, color, and thickness. Though you've handled your equipment innumerable times over your lifetime, have you ever stopped to examine it? Sure you know what feels good, but experiment with varying touch (and kiss and tongue) techniques to find out what really tickles your fancy.

The *shaft,* which extends from the base just above the scrotum, is connected to the head and gets hard as the two tubular structures (corpora cavernosa) within it fill with blood during erection.

The *head* bulges with sensitivity and nerves at the very top of the shaft. Its swollen appearance is a result of the widening of the spongy tissue of the corpus spongiosom that surrounds the urethra.

The *urethral meatus* is the hole at the top of the head through which urine and ejaculate are expelled (though not at the same time).

The *frenulum* is one of the most important pleasure spots on the entire male body. This small notch of connective tissue on the underside of the shaft just below the head attaches the foreskin to the penis.

The *corona* is the swollen ridge of tissue that surrounds the base of the head. A highly sensitive area, some evolutionary psychologists theorize that this bulge is designed to expunge the sperm of other men or sexual rivals.

The *foreskin* is the double layer of protective skin that is sometimes removed when the man is still a baby through a process called *circumcision.*

The *prostate* is often compared to the female G-spot and is located between the bladder and the pelvic floor against the front wall of his anus. Composed of smooth muscle fibers, tissue, tubes, and glands, it produces the milky white fluid that helps to carry and sustain sperm.

The testes are contained within the *scrotal sac,* which hangs below the body at a temperature of one or two degrees cooler than regular body temperature to promote sperm production. The scrotum is comprised of thin, soft muscles, and each testicle is connected to a spermatic cord.

DR. JESS SAYS . . .

Penises can and do break, so handle them with care! The tunica albuginea, which surrounds the corpora cavernosa, can rupture when the penis is erect. This is a medical emergency that often requires surgery, so get over your embarrassment and seek medical attention immediately. Though not particularly common, penile fractures can result from slamming the head of the penis against a hard surface (like a pelvic bone or coccyx) or forceful bending.

DOES SIZE MATTER?
Yes. But not in the way you might think.

Size matters—but mostly in terms of finding the right fit, and bigger is not necessarily better. In fact, though a longer penis may afford you greater bragging rights in the locker room, it can actually be a mixed blessing in the bedroom. Some of us have longer vaginas and some of us have shorter ones, but the vast majority of women report being perfectly satisfied with their partner's size. When it comes to pleasure, women say they're more likely to prefer a wider penis to a longer one. This is no surprise given that the length of the average vagina is shorter than that of the average penis.

If you're still not convinced, the research backs this up. Only 6 percent of women rate their partner's penis size as small, and 84 percent say they're "very satisfied" with their lover's size. In contrast, only 55 percent of men report a similar level of satisfaction with their own size. Studies that assess the average length of an erect penis

tend to vary in their conclusions, but a review of fifty studies that included 11,531 penises reveals a combined average of 5.5–6.3 inches (with an average circumference of 4.7–5.1 inches). Some men are growers and others are showers: A smaller flaccid penis will grow considerably more than a larger one, resulting in less of a size differential once they're both hard. For this reason, flaccid size is not a good indicator of erect length. Moreover, the size of a penis is entirely unrelated to one's capacity to experience pleasure, arousal and orgasm.

Though junk mail campaigns suggest that the penile enlargement industry is booming, the reality is that most of these products and procedures are useless. Urologist Dr. Aaron Blumenfeld, MD, FRCS(C), explains:

"There are many pills, creams, or machines that may advertise a way to improve this, but for the most part, they are all bogus. So what does work? Weight loss might, as it allows more of the flaccid penis to be visible. Surgeries are a last resort, as they are high-risk and can only improve length to a minimal degree. Many people are dissatisfied with the cosmetic results post-operatively."

As for the rumors suggesting that foot or hand size is indicative of penis size, we now have evidence to refute this myth. Big feet equal big shoes and that's about it.

FAQ: WHY DOES MY PENIS KEEP DRIPPING AFTER I PEE?

This is a common complaint from many men, and there is a perfectly sound anatomical explanation: Because your internal urethral sphincter, the muscle that automatically pinches the pee hole closed, is located several inches away from the tip of your penis, some urine gets trapped on the other side. A few shakes may help to empty it out, or you can try running your finger along the underside of your penis (base to tip) to draw out the remaining liquid.

ALL ABOUT EJACULATE

There seems to be a considerable amount of misinformation floating around about ejaculate, its contents, and the supposed benefits of swallowing. From "cookbooks" touting semen as a cure-all for disease to men's magazines celebrating swallowing as the antidote to depression, it can be difficult to differentiate between fact and fantasy. Let's set the record straight.

Ejaculate is primarily composed of water but also contains small amounts of fructose, vitamin C, magnesium, zinc, potassium, and sodium bicarbonate. Though one load of ejaculate contains over 200 million sperm, they are so tiny that they account for only approximately 2 percent of total ejaculate volume. The amount of semen ejaculated usually increases slightly with longer periods of abstinence, but on average men release about a half-teaspoon of fluid at a time. The volume of one's semen is not necessarily an indicator of virility or fertility but rather how much time has elapsed since his last ejaculation.

Urologists believe that the taste of semen tends to be relatively constant, as it contains the requisite ingredients to support the survival of sperm; however, anecdotal reports from men and women who have tasted ejaculate suggest otherwise. Many experienced tasters believe that eating sweet fruits, vegetables, and herbs can temper the taste of semen and heighten its sugary flavor. They also suggest that smoking and ingesting caffeine and preservatives can result in a more bitter taste.

Human sperm can live on surfaces until they dry out, but detergent and soap kill them on contact by stripping them of their cell membrane. Fresh water also kills sperm due to the process of osmotic shock, but water cannot be used to kill sperm in the vagina or reproductive tract.

FOR SEX GEEKS

"Shrinkage" is not a myth. Changes in blood flow in response to temperature are to blame. But don't worry. The change is a function of the sympathetic nervous system and is only temporary.

FAQ: SINCE I EJACULATE THROUGH THE SAME HOLE THAT I PEE OUT OF, WHAT STOPS THE PEE FROM COMING OUT WHEN I ORGASM? AND WHY IS IT SO HARD TO PEE AFTER SEX?

Dr. Aaron Blumenfeld explains that during sexual stimulation, "parasympathetic neural pathways are activated, causing an erection to occur. At the time of orgasm, sympathetic neural pathways cause an increase in the pressure of the urinary sphincter and bladder neck and cause the muscular contractions of ejaculation. This ensures that the ejaculate isn't pushed into the bladder [and urine isn't pushed out]. Postorgasm, the sympathetic receptors in the prostate are still partially stimulated, increasing the resistance at the bladder neck and inhibiting the ability of the bladder to contract, making it harder to pee."

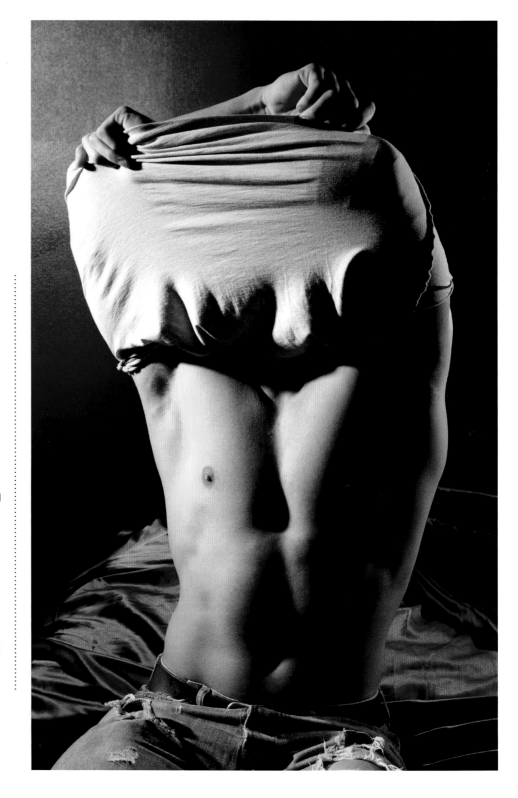

UNCOVER HIS EROGENOUS ZONES

We often reduce male pleasure to the penis and assume that anything goes when it comes to sexually satisfying a man, but nothing could be further from the truth. Men are highly sexual beings with unique personal tastes, and you can discover new pleasure zones and techniques at any age. As you experiment with new erogenous zones, cover his eyes with a blindfold to heighten his physical experience through sensory deprivation.

Perineum

This stretch of skin between the balls and the anus may be the hottest spot on his body. Not only can you massage his inner penis through his perineum (also known as the "taint" and "gooch"), but sweeping your hands over it during orgasm can produce a rush of pleasure throughout his body as his prostate responds to your firm touch.

Raphe

This is the dividing line that runs all the way from the anus to the tip of his cock, passing over the perineum, scrotum, and shaft. Stick your tongue all the way out and trace it over this supersensitive spot to tease him into your mouth.

Treasure Trail

The space between his belly button and his pubic mound is highly sensitive to light touch, and its proximity to his pelvic region encourages blood flow to all the right places. Tongue a line down his lower abs to the top of his pubic mound and then trace the outline of his cock with your tongue.

Nipples

Women's nipples tend to get a lot of attention since they're at the center of their breasts, but this area can have orgasmic potential in men, too! Twirl your tongue around this sensitive spot during foreplay or nibble playfully on them while he's coming to spread his orgasmic sensations from his genitals to his chest.

Ankles

Reflexologists consider the indentations below the inner and outer ankles to be sources of stimulation for the penis, prostate, and testes. Clasp his lower ankles between your thumbs and middle fingers while in the 69 position, or offer him a foot rub to help him unwind after a long hard day.

Inner Thighs

The complex intersection of nerve endings in this area coupled with the anticipation built as you near his penis make the inner thighs a top erogenous zone for most men. Touch him between his legs when out in public, allowing the back of your hand to briefly brush against his cock. Trickle your fingertips from the top of his knee up to the apex of his thighs while you suck him into your mouth later that night.

Shoulders

The pressure points in the middle of the tendons on either side of his neck often hold tension that can inhibit both his physical and subjective sexual response. Help him to relax and get his head into the game by gently kneading your thumbs in circular motions around this tender area.

PERSONAL PLEASURE MAP

Traditional body mapping research involves recognizing areas of the body in which emotions are felt and processed. Finnish researchers have found that when asked to describe where they experienced different emotions in their bodies, participants' responses are fairly constant—even across cultures. For example, happiness creates feelings across the entire body whereas fear activates feelings in the chest. Since sex involves both physical and emotional responses, mapping your pleasure out for both you and your partner can enhance the experience in both your body and mind.

Over the years, you've gotten to know your body better than anyone else ever will, so show off that knowledge and show her exactly how and where you like to be touched. Use the diagram below as a personal pleasure map, and feel free to make changes or redo this exercise a few times per year as your tastes and reactions change.

Color each area according to your preferences:

Yellow indicates you enjoy a soft, gentle caress or kiss of the area.

Blue suggests that you prefer a firm touch or fondle.

Green demarcates the regions where you like a wetter, deeper kiss.

Purple shows the spots that desire ...

(You fill in the blank.)

Red areas are off-limits to all touch.

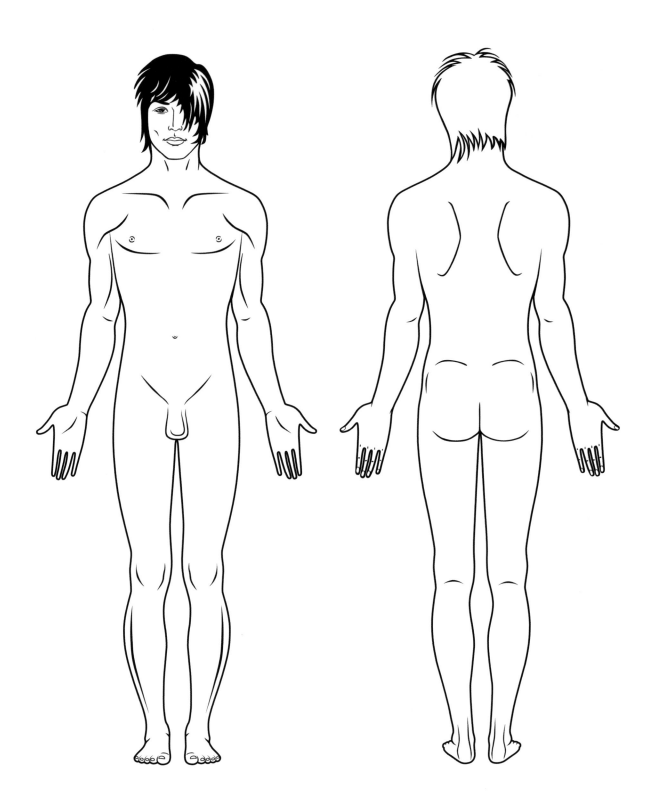

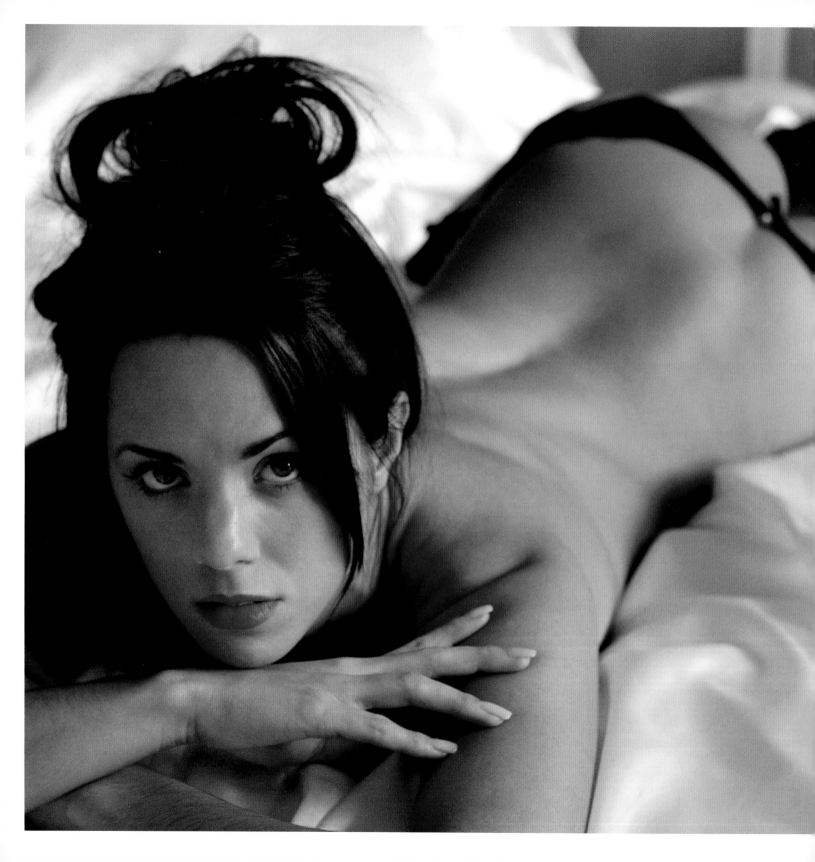

02 *Desire and Seduction*

Desire is fundamental to hot sex. Without it, sex is a mere *act* as opposed to an *experience*. When you are teeming with desire and drunk with lust, your senses are heightened and your orgasmic response intensified. When you first meet a new partner or potential lover, feelings of desire overtake you as the period of limerence unfolds. Thoughts of your lover or lover to-be are persistent, intrusive, and involuntary. With time, the connection intensifies and the carnal thoughts subside. Respect, care, and tenderness increase and often the craving for sex slackens even as your attraction remains high. Despite this falloff in natural sexual tension, studies show that sex is most satisfying in long-term relationships.

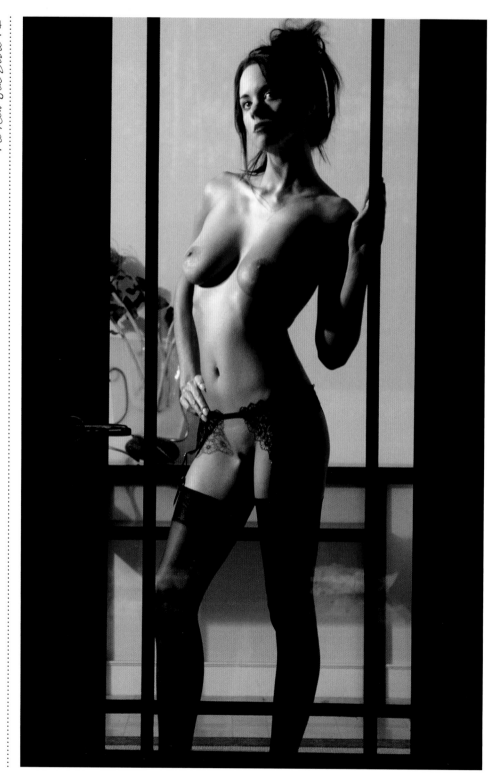

MAKE YOUR LOVER CRAVE YOU

Desire and seduction go hand in hand and both are fundamental to hot sex. Though your levels of desire are impacted by many factors (diet, stress, sleep, and exercise to name just a few), skillful sexual seduction can attenuate the impact of these lifestyle factors. Similarly, when you are overcome by untamed desire, you become naturally inspired to seduce your lover in new and compelling ways. Neither desire nor seduction can flourish into sexual pleasure without the other, and both are prerequisites to every fulfilling sexual encounter.

Whether you've been lovers for five months or five years—or fifty!—maintaining the spark and making your lover crave you is well worth the effort, for both sexual and emotional fulfillment. Here are a few strategies to make your lover ache for you.

Be playful! Tap into your inner child. Studies suggest that playfulness may be a sign of maturity, and a sense of humor ranks as the most important character trait sought in a long-term partner. Take time to play together as you would have in your early years: Hit up the swing set at your local park, visit the zoo or an amusement park without the kids, go for a swim at sunset, or watch a movie from the backseat at a drive-in theater. And try to work some playfulness into your daily routines, too. Flash him a glimpse of your thong while you're in the kitchen, or press your cock into her backside while cleaning up after breakfast to leave her aching for more all day long.

Brush up on your skills. Even if you are the best lover your sweetheart has ever met, you can always learn new techniques and approaches to supplement your current repertoire. Who can resist a nighttime "practice" session?

Switch roles between the boardroom (or kitchen table) and the bedroom. The fantasy of having a lady/gentleman in the street but a freak in the sheets is a common one, so showcase your most refined manners in public and draw out your most primal urges once the lights are lowered. The anticipation might just make your lover pull over on the way home to sample what's to come.

Maintain separate interests, hobbies, and social groups. Autonomy has been shown to be connected to higher levels of pleasure, satisfaction, and orgasm in both men and women. In one study 39 percent of respondents reported that they have a healthier relationship because they maintain some degree of independence from their partner. Time apart can actually create sexual tension, as your brain responds to the mystery of your absence and novelty of your return. Maintaining your own interests outside of your relationship also breeds curiosity, which can trigger chemical and brain reactions similar to those experienced during the exciting early stages of your relationship.

Take on multiple personalities in bed. Being a submissive damsel in distress may help to draw out his inner macho dominant, but switching things up will keep him guessing and coming back for more. Even if you prefer to submit to his every need, be sure to surprise him once in a while by initiating sex, taking control, and letting him lie back and indulge in the prowess of your inner dominant.

Indulge your lover in her fantasies. If she fantasizes about being ravaged by two strangers in the backseat of her car, tease her with tidbits of this fantasy during flirting and sex play. Whisper in her ear, "I want to share you," or drive her to a secluded spot and blindfold her as you talk her into believing that you're a total stranger. Supporting her in her most intense fantasies will entrench your role in her sexual script and intensify your erotic bond.

Encourage your honey to cheat … but only in his mind. Sharing your partner may be the furthest thing from your sexual radar, but encouraging your lover to fantasize about other people and scenarios can plant the seed for a lifetime of scintillating sex. Our fantasies are often moderated by culturally enforced inhibitions and expectations, including a focus on monogamy. By giving your lover permission to fantasize about scenarios you might never live out, you will inevitably broaden his sexual horizons and encourage shared fantasies to deepen your connection. Feed his fantasies by telling him how much they turn you on and try to find common ground. If he fantasizes about having a threesome with another lady, have fun admiring other women in public and describe to him in detail exactly what turns you on: "I love her tits. I bet you'd like to watch me kiss them." "I've never kissed a girl, but her lips look so luscious."

Talk dirty. This is the ultimate sexual skill, and it is most effective if you throw it into the mix hours (or even days) ahead of time. Talking dirty in bed is hot, but utilizing dirty talk outside of the bedroom establishes the foundation for rapturous desire and mind-blowing sex. (Look ahead to Chapter 3 for some dirty talk ideas.)

Play the bad boy (or girl) once in a while. Research suggests that risk-takers are highly attractive as lovers but not as long-term partners. Being a sweetheart will keep her happy outside of the bedroom, but once you're behind closed doors, let your naughty side shine.

Cuddle naked. The connection fostered through skin-to-skin contact involves a complex interplay of chemical reactions in the body and mind. Cuddling is not only erotic and intimate, but for men, it is positively correlated with happiness levels.

Wear red. This is an easy one and the attraction to color is actually grounded in research. Not only is this bright hue associated with love, passion, and sex, but also studies suggest that both men and women are more attracted to the opposite sex when they're wearing red. One group of researchers compared women's reactions to photographs of men set against red and white backgrounds and found that the men with red surroundings were consistently rated as more attractive. However, when heterosexual men participated in the same study, the color of the backdrop had no bearing on attractiveness ratings, suggesting that the allure of the color red is related to the sexual as opposed to merely the aesthetic. Other research suggests that men are also more attracted to women in red and are drawn to both red clothing and lipstick.

HOW TO GET IN THE MOOD (AND STAY THERE)

We often assume that attraction and arousal are physical. However, as desire originates in our minds, both attraction and arousal are, in fact, cognitive. While *physical* arousal and desire might flow freely with ease, sometimes *mental* arousal, which is reliant on our state of mind, can be thwarted by intrusive thoughts. Whether you're worried about a big presentation the next day, a disagreement you had with a friend, or ongoing financial woes, nonsexual thoughts can extinguish sexual arousal or impede sexual satisfaction.

While there may be times you want your lover to think about baseball or dinner to keep from climaxing, most of the time you want to focus your attention on what's to come or the task at hand. If intrusive thoughts are getting in the way, try these approaches to managing them.

Relax. Take time to relax your mind and body before jumping into sexual activity. Give each other a massage, read a few pages of erotica, dance the lambada or rumba, meditate together, or take a jog outdoors together, if that calms your mood. Fantasize or daydream about an appealing scenario—sexual or otherwise.

Just breathe. Practice slow and purposeful breathing, focusing solely on the flow of air in and out of your lungs. Breathe in through your nose and out through your mouth.

Tune in to your body. Wear a blindfold or close your eyes and touch yourself, focusing only on the physical sensations. When your sensations are sufficiently aroused, go ahead and bring yourself to climax, call in your partner to finish the job, or pause and go about your day, leaving yourself craving sexual fulfillment later on.

Be dismissive. Allow the thoughts to flow in and out of your mind freely. You cannot force unwanted thoughts to disappear entirely, so if that unfinished tax return pops into your mind during fellatio, acknowledge it and let it go.

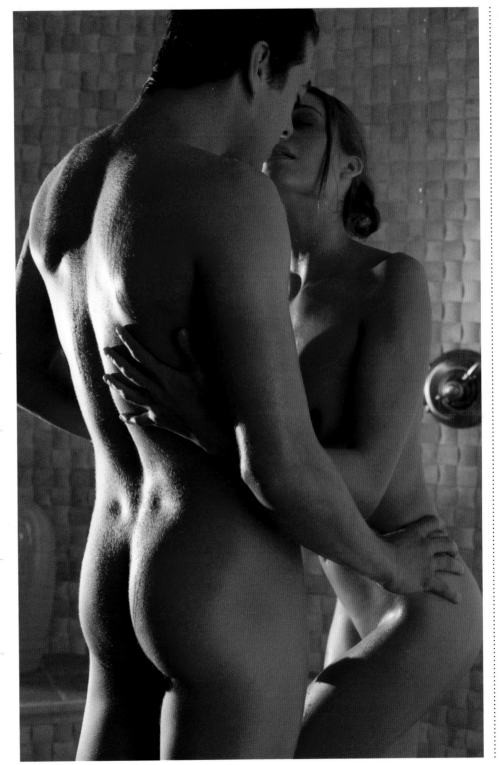

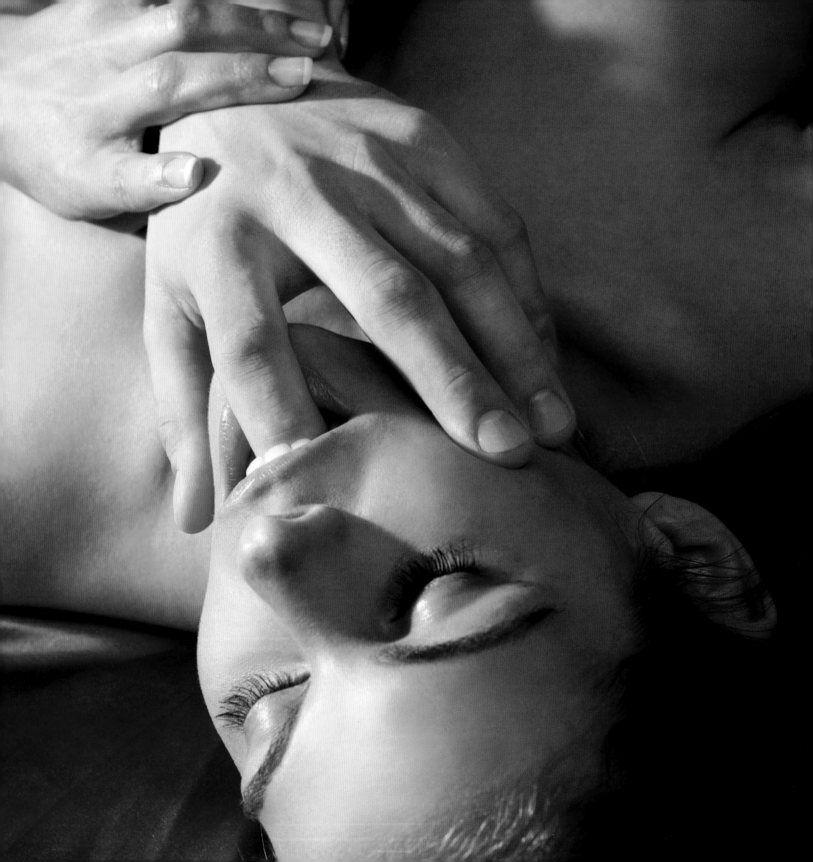

EROTIC TOUCH

Physical affection may be the most powerful of all love languages, and we have come to associate intimate touch with deep commitment. Women rate affection as one of the most important components of a loving relationship.

Plus, researchers have found that couples who caress one another experience a reduction in stress hormones, blood pressure, and blood sugar alongside an increase in oxytocin levels, improved pulmonary functioning, and heightened immunity. On top of the purported health benefits, being touched by a loved one also feels great!

Erotic touch is an extension of loving touch and different from therapeutic touch. You don't need to work out the knots in her back or soothe his aching neck during an erotic encounter. Instead, your touch is intended for mutual pleasure, relaxation, and connection, and it may or may not lead to further sex play.

Unfortunately, many couples allow their erotic touch to taper off as their relationship progresses, and women often complain that their lovers do not touch or hug them in nonsexual situations. This is a shame, as intimate touch is not just a precursor to sex but is related to higher levels of relationship satisfaction. Learning to touch your lover's entire body is a simple way to boost your happiness and ignite your sex life, so take some time to slow down and explore your bodies in their entirety without rushing to the genitals for instant gratification.

Massage Techniques

The sensual massage techniques that follow will have your lover's body writhing in pleasure and impassioned desire. Before you begin, make sure the room is a comfortable temperature and your partner is relaxed, whether that means sitting in a chair or lying on the bed. Make it interesting by giving her a blindfold to wear. You can take turns massaging each other, or dedicate an entire session to worshipping your lover's body alone.

Spider pulls are the perfect way to draw awareness and blood to the surface of her skin. Start with your fingers outstretched and the pads of your fingertips resting gently against her skin. Slowly and gently pull all five fingers together into the center with the lightest touch possible.

FOR SEX GEEKS

The fingertips are among the most reactive erogenous zones during arousal. Your heavy breathing cleanses carbon dioxide from the blood and alters the ionic balance of bodily fluids. The result is an increase in nerve activity and excitation, which results in tingling at the skin's surface—particularly at the fingertips.

Raindrops produce a tingling sensation as you gently flutter the pads of your fingertips along his most sensitive regions. Start with his spine, underarms, shoulder blades, and butt cheeks.

Finger stripes allow you to draw erotic energy to a focused area of her body. Cover all five fingers in oil and run them in a straight line down the backs of her thighs, inner arms, or abdomen. Then retrace your path using your middle knuckles.

Palm circles get the blood flowing to all the right places. Just be sure to cover your hands in a light massage oil before circling them over his chest, abs, and hips.

Figure eights allow you to explore her body with large sweeping sensations. Use two wet fingers to trace loops of figure-eight patterns along her collarbone, arms, and the sides of her breasts.

Tongue trails offer a reminder that you don't need your hands to give a sensual massage. Trace your tongue all around his hot spots, alternating between a pointed tip and a wide, flat tongue.

The body slide is an advanced technique common in high-end massage parlors. Your lover lies on his stomach and you slide your entire body down the full length of his backside. You'll need to slather yourselves in oil for this one!

Awakening touch uses only the backs of your fingernails. This activates the nerve endings, referred to as the *tactile corpuscles*, that are most sensitive to light touch and are primed for heightened pleasure, as they don't interpret pain.

Temperature play can be highly erotic as you shift between breathing warm air against the skin with a wide open mouth and cool air with tightly pursed lips to activate your lover's sensitive thermo-receptors.

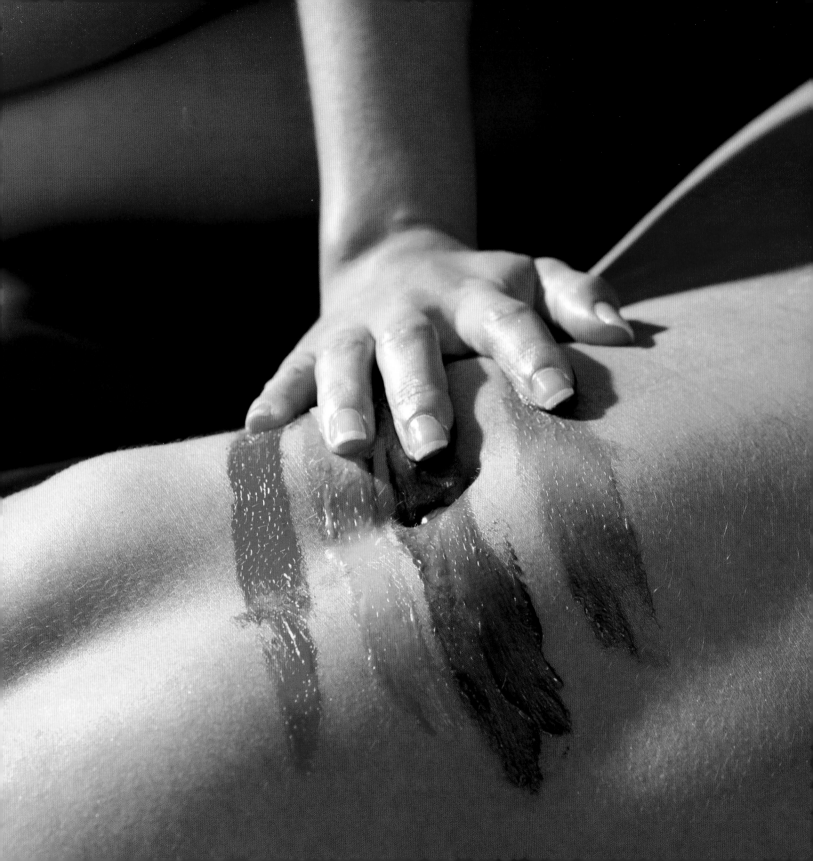

A SEXOLOGIST'S GUIDE TO KISSING

Though kissing may be a deeply entrenched dating and mating ritual in our culture, many cultures have prospered without locking lips, which serves as a reminder that kissing is an erotic art (as opposed to a reproductive imperative).

Making out results in a flurry of feel-good hormones that promote relaxation and bonding. Yet the sexes view it differently. Men are more likely than women to seek and initiate deep-tongue kissing, and they tend to utilize it as a means to an end (sex), whereas many women report that they view kissing as a barometer with which to gauge their lover's commitment and monitor their relationship status.

However you view it, smooching plays a prominent role in seduction, romantic attachment, and sexual arousal. Unfortunately in long-term relationships, we often stop kissing or push passionate kissing aside in favor of other forms of foreplay. And while there is no universal hierarchy of sex acts, research suggests that kissing is not only good for your health but also promotes happier relationships. In one study conducted by behavioral scientist Kerry Floyd, couples who were instructed to kiss more often reported fewer fights, greater relationship satisfaction, less stress, and lower cholesterol in comparison to couples who received no instruction with regard to kissing.

Despite the mounting evidence that getting to first base is good for you and your love life, keeping things fresh can be a challenge. Grab your partner and try the following suggestions and techniques designed to keep you happy, healthy, and very much in love for years to come.

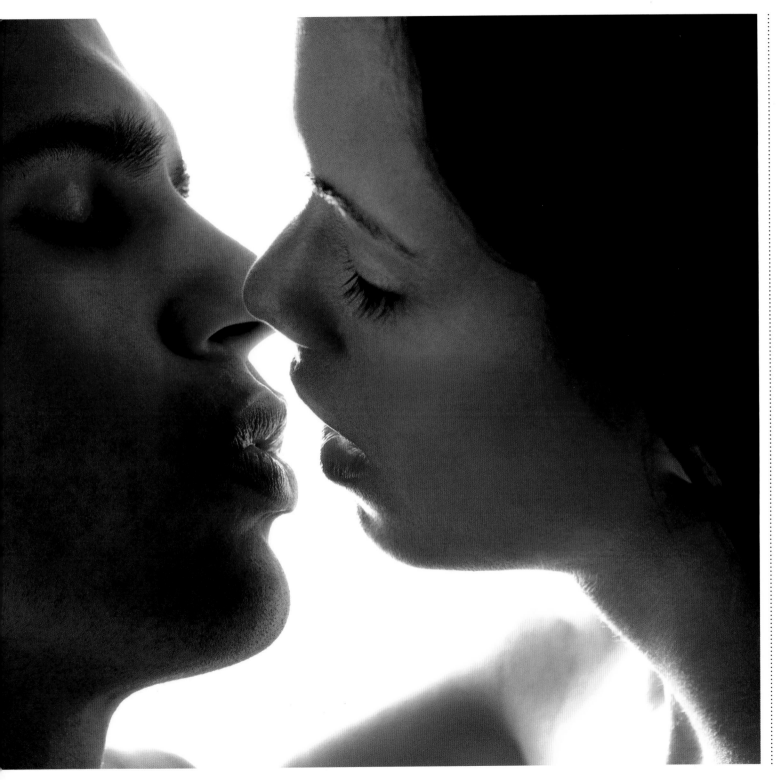

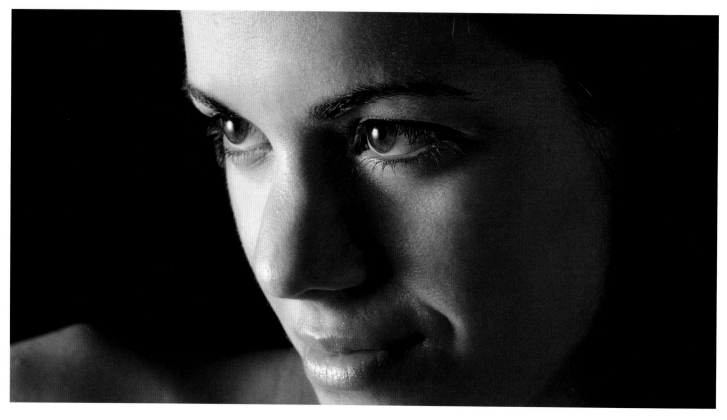

The Soft-Lipped Kiss

Some people believe that the world is divided into two types of kissers: soft-lipped and firm-lipped. But the reality is that our sexual style varies according to our mood just as our appetite changes from day to day. If your lover seeks romance and often needs help relaxing to get in the mood, slide your lips gently against his with only featherlight contact. Take your time and gently pucker his lower lip between your lips, allowing your easy breathing to slow his breath rate and send his body into a state of deep relaxation.

Lip Lining

Give your honey a peek into your oral skills as you masterfully trace your tongue around the curves of her lips, paying extra attention to the thin skin in the corners where the upper and lower lips meet. If her lips remain closed, sensually slide your tongue from one side to the other just inside the crease.

Sweet Spot

You're probably familiar with the frenulum of the penis, but this sensitive connective tissue also exists just inside the lips. Slide your tongue inside and twirl it purposefully around the shallow space between his upper lips and teeth before moving on to deep, French kissing.

Basic Tongue Twirl

As you press your lips together, tilt your head slightly to the side and suck gently as you twirl your tongue around hers.

Top-Shelf Kiss

Swipe your tongue along the roof of your lover's mouth, a sensitive and oft-neglected area.

Code Word

Kiss your lover out in public at every stoplight, or come up with a code word (e.g., *thank you* or *fun*) and stop what you're doing to French kiss whenever you hear this buzzword.

Facial

Hold one another by the cheeks as you kiss deeply and passionately. The face is the most sensual part of the body but receives little attention in the way of touch.

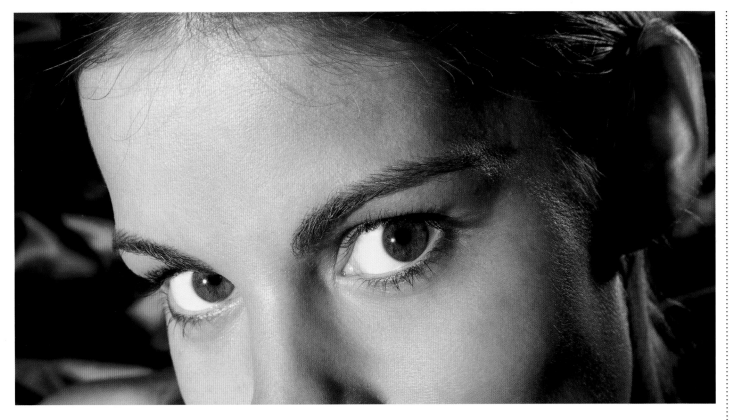

HOW TO FLIRT WITH YOUR LOVER

Flirting may be an art, but it is also a custom that is universal across cultures. Not only is flirting essential to human reproduction, but evolutionary psychologists suggest that humans owe our advanced civilization and technological developments to this fine courtship skill.

Our ancestors used body language, eye contact, and verbal cues to charm one another and send signals with regard to sexual interest. Today, we express our attraction to one another using a similar set of subtle (and not so subtle) prompts designed to take the place of awkward conversations. Rather than walking up to a stranger and asking if our attraction is mutual, we utilize an array of signals ranging from shy smiles to licking lips to convey our desire. When we first meet a potential lover, flirting often comes naturally as we feel compelled to express both our desire and our longing to *be desired*.

In long-term relationships, however, our ancient primal brain often gives way to other parts that are wired for reason and executive functioning. Flirting becomes less of a necessity as we communicate our needs in more concrete terms, often using language.

That said, flirting is essential to keeping the sexual spark alive, as it draws sex out of the bedroom and into our daily routines and eroticizes the relationship. By teasing and tantalizing your lover in nonsexual situations, you prime her mind and body for sex at a later time. Flirting isn't about being the life of the party, the one that everyone in attendance wants to go home with. It's about meaningful clues between two people that signal, "I want *you*." If it's been a while since you actually flirted with your partner, or if you've ever felt that you're just "not good" at it, here are some tips for flirting:

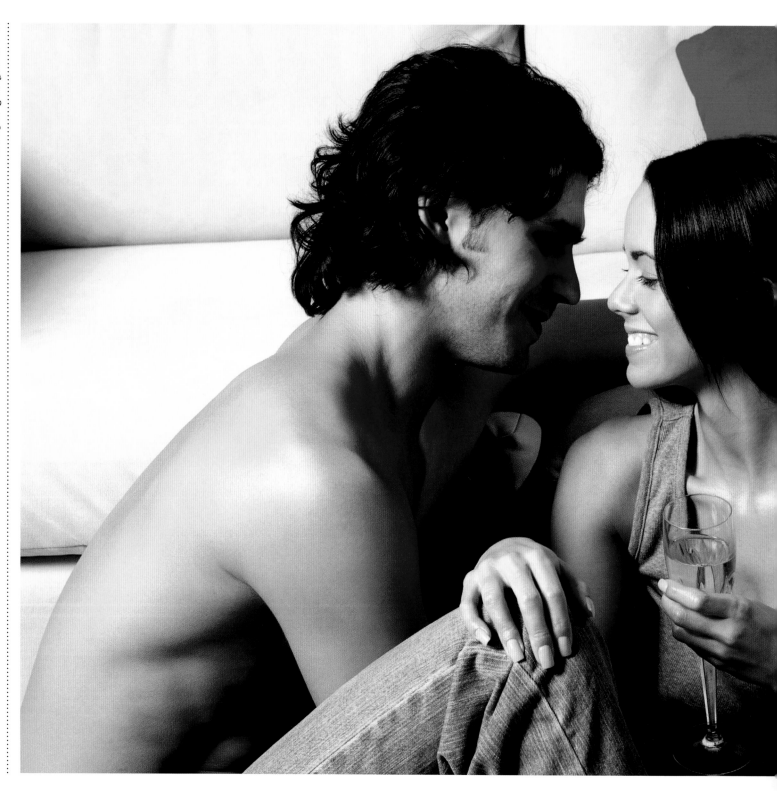

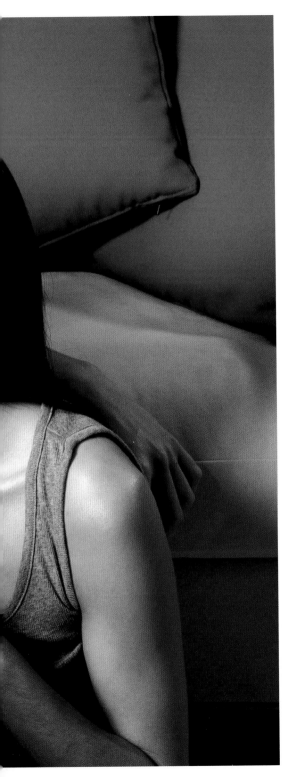

Touch suggestively when out in public. Leave the groping and PDA for the teenagers. A peck on the cheek or a quick brush of the thighs can go a long way to building sexual tension.

Be boastful. Compliment and revere your lover in group situations. This social signal reinforces your attraction and bond.

Make eye contact at unexpected times. Sit across from one another at a party or gathering and sneak a coy smile as you lower your eyes. Fall back on the old standby—a wink—when you think no one is looking. The thought of having "gotten away with" something, especially if you're at a fancy function, can send sparks of desire in your lover.

Be covert. Use a secret code word or phrase to indicate your thirst for intimacy or sex. Make it a silly word and have fun by working it in to conversations with other people. "Oh, you have a dog! My husband would love to own a *rhinoceros*."

Take a cue from the animal kingdom. Research suggests that our pick-up cues are only slightly more sophisticated than those of animals. Women signal their interest through giggles, soft laughs, and hair twirling while men respond by arching their bodies and leaning back, much like a bird puffing out its chest. To show themselves as the best possible mate for breeding, peacocks show off their beautiful plumage, camels work up a mouthful of lather, and deer rack their antlers. Create a signature look, accessory, or gesture that's just between you. If it's a particular pair of earrings, give one a tug when you know he's watching you. If it's leaving that five-o'clock stubble linger past midnight, let it be a gentle reminder of how that stubble is going to feel between her thighs.

SEDUCTION TECHNIQUES

If flirting sets the stage for establishing mutual sexual desire, seduction pulls back the curtain to reveal the enticing opening act. Accordingly, seduction is not a precursor to but rather an integral component of sex. It establishes the tone of the entire encounter and helps you to get your head into the game before your bodies even touch.

The way you seduce your partner greatly impacts the path and outcome of each sexual experience. The sneaky "poke" from behind or a fumbled "Want to have sex?" may convey the same message as an effusive display of desire but will seldom produce the same response. For many of us (and women in particular), our erotic scripts, the stories and attitudes that fuel sexual desire involve the experience of being desired. For this reason, the most masterful seducers are those who can convey their sexual desire in the most genuine, discernible, and believable of ways.

From straightforward expressions to suggestive nuance, seduction is an art—not a science—so it's up to you to create your own masterpiece.

COMPLIMENTS WILL GET YOU EVERYWHERE

Compliments are gifts of love and among the greatest sources of motivation, as most of us enjoy having our egos stroked as much as we like having our most sensitive body parts stroked. Research suggests that compliments are as motivating as cash rewards, but the benefits associated with compliments go both ways, as the receiver experiences a bump in self-esteem while the giver gets a natural mood boost. Learning to receive compliments graciously with a simple thank-you or smile is just as important as doling them out.

There are different approaches to the compliment, and it's wise to find a balance between compliments of pleasantry, flirtation, and seduction. Compliments of pleasantry refer to those that we might pay to friends, family, and acquaintances: "You look nice today." "I like your shoes." "Nice haircut." Flirtatious compliments are intended to express erotic interest: "You look hot." "Your legs look amazing." "You're so beautiful." Seductive compliments tap into our animalistic desire and primal urges, serving as a solicitation of sex, though not necessarily in the immediate future: "I want to tear your clothes off." "You make me want to bend you over and make you scream." "I want to hold you down and watch your body quiver with pleasure."

Weaving pleasant, flirtatious, and seductive compliments into your daily routine can work wonders for your sex life. "That's a nice skirt. It accentuates the curves of your ass. It's going to look even better when it's pushed up around your waist as I drive my cock into you."

You can also use compliments in bed to intensify arousal:

"I love when you . . ."

"You're the best at . . ."

"It drives me wild when . . ."

"I can't resist your . . ."

SURPRISE SEDUCTION

Predictability is the perfect recipe for boredom in the bedroom. As our brains and bodies become accustomed to routine, the excitement automatically subsides. Initiating sex at an unexpected moment during a shared nonsexual activity can help to stave off boredom due to predictability. The next time you're watching TV, doing the dishes, or cooking a meal, see if you can stealthily arouse your lover. Graze the back of your hand against her neck or cop a feel from behind. Be persistent. Not everyone responds to interruptions of routines in an immediately positive manner, so let your lover know just how hard you're willing to work to get him onto the dining room table or bend her over the kitchen counter.

SEXTING

Sex and technology form the perfect pair to enhance your love life. Sending sexy texts throughout the day or week can cause tension to mount to levels at which you'll want to tear one another's clothes off. Some sexting tips:

Ask first. Sending unsolicited sexts is tantamount to harassment, so ask your flirty friend if she wants your pics and suggestive tête-à-tête before you send them. Permission can be sexy (she'll wonder what you have up your sleeve), so use your imagination and be seductive and playful.

Leave something to the imagination. If the first photo you send is a hot shot of your entire body or genitals, you leave no space for buildup and anticipation. Make sexting about teasing, so that the grand finale (you in person) is even hotter. Take a shot of something that's significant for you—the back of your knees, for example, because you love it when he blows on them. An added bonus: If he opens his message at work or if the kids get a hold of his phone, there's not a lot of uncomfortable explaining.

Be referential, rather than direct. Instead of sexting, "I loved sucking you off last night," try something more subtle: "Tonight is MY turn." He knows what you mean, and he's likely going to follow up the first chance he gets.

Ax emoticons. Want to ruin a perfectly hot sext like "I want to taste you"? Add an animated winky face to expertly kill the mood.

SET THE MOOD

Candles, flowers, and heels are not cliché. They're the perfect props to set the scene for a sensual evening. We often make efforts to create an erotic space during the early stages of a relationship but neglect to do so as time passes, so be sure to revisit your inner romantic even after years of marriage: Play the song from your first date or kiss, visit a location that reminds you of your first date, or surprise your lover with a bottle of chocolate syrup and a paintbrush to inspire some erotic creativity.

Because sex involves all five senses, including sounds, textures, lighting, scents, and even tastes into your seduction routine can overwhelm your lover—in the best of ways. Some people are easily distracted by sounds, so music or even a white noise machine may help to keep your lover focused on the action as opposed to worrying about what is happening next door. For others, lighting is essential to increasing body confidence while others feel sexiest when their skin is set against soft, lush fabrics.

Even the temperature can affect the mood when it comes to sex. Research suggests that warmer temperatures are conducive to orgasm, as they promote blood flow that is essential to orgasm. One study, at the University of Groningen, found that cold feet can be a significant hindrance to arousal and a cozy pair of socks increases the chances of orgasm from 50 percent to 80 percent for women.

LONG-DISTANCE LUST

Absence makes the heart grow fonder and the groin ache with delight. When you live together and have easy access to one another, the novelty can fade, so recreating a scenario in which you must pine for your lover can be an effective seduction technique. Use a video phone call program to call your honey midday and offer a taste of what's to come. Unbutton your shirt for a quick one-minute teaser, but then come home late to heighten the tension and make your lover wait. Or go completely retro and write your inamorata a love letter of all the things you'd like to do to her when she's finished reading it.

HIGH SCHOOL SWEETHEARTS

Set a rule that you cannot have sex in your house for two weeks. This will force you to get creative and find new places to get it on. Get freaky in the car, a public washroom, a department store fitting room, the park at night, a movie theater, or even in your own backyard. The thrill of getting caught not only harkens back to your younger (and perhaps wilder days) but can also activate the flight-or-fight response that heightens your senses and intensifies pleasure.

LEAVE YOUR TOYS OUT!

If you have difficulty initiating sex, leaving out a book, toy, blindfold, or other prop can signal your desire and spark your lover's interest. You may also want to pique their curiosity in more subtle ways: Leave a pair of crotchless panties by his briefcase, drop a poem in her lunch box, or replace his bookmark with a sexy photo.

Though toys and props are often enjoyed in pairs, there is nothing in the rule book prohibiting you from getting a head start. You may even want to wait until your lover is just minutes away from home before busting out your favorite toy and getting warmed up. Stage your private session in an opportune location so that your lover gets a sexy surprise when they walk in the door. Give them a warm welcome by inviting them to join in on the fun...

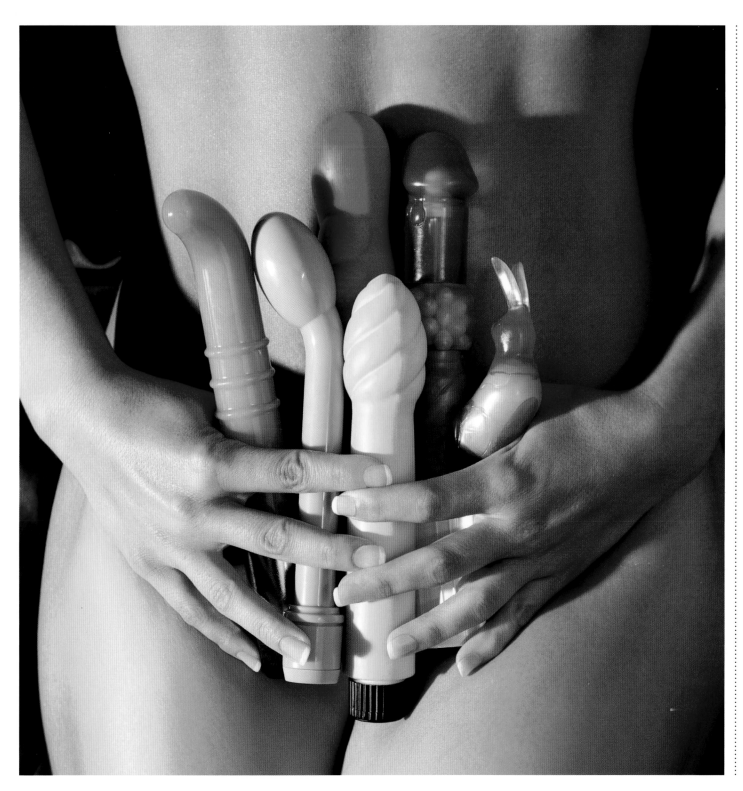

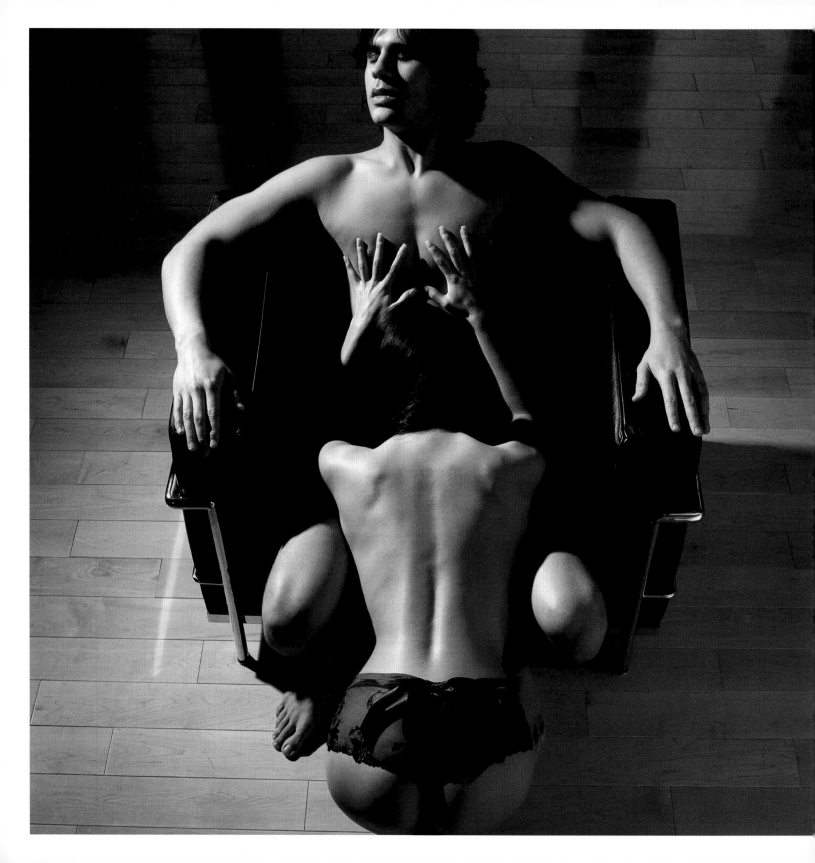

03 Sizzling Oral Sex: The Hottest Finger, Lips, and Tongue Techniques

If you're eager to get a jump on some scorching oral sex secrets, then turn to page 70 (for her) and 80 (for him). And if you want to brush up your sexy trash talk, turn to page 68. However, I'd be remiss if I didn't include that most basic of oral activity—talking—in this chapter.

HOT ORAL: HOW TO TALK TO YOUR LOVER ABOUT SEX

Conversations about sex are seldom easy, but open communication is fundamental to a more satisfying sex life. While in almost every other realm, talking the talk is easier than walking the walk, sex seems to be the exception. Research actually suggests that people are more comfortable *having* sex than *talking* about it. This communication gap not only wreaks havoc on our sex lives, but it also takes a toll on our intimacy levels, expressions of affection, and overall relationships.

HIGHLIGHT THE POSITIVE

As you open conversations about sex, highlight the positive and begin with lighter topics. Start by talking about what you already enjoy about your sex life and offer compliments whenever possible. Ideally, your comfort levels will increase and sex talk will become a regular part of your interactions as opposed to awkward discussions you have when you encounter problems in your sex life. By spending some time talking about the positive elements of your sex life, you normalize sexual conversations as constructive and ongoing as opposed to reactionary.

Here are a few lines to get you started with positive sex talk:

"I love when you . . ."

"One thing that I really like is . . ."

"You're the best at . . ."

"Do you remember that time at the theater when you . . . ? That felt so good!"

ASK LEADING QUESTIONS

Asking questions to learn more about your lover's needs is another effective approach to improving your sexual communication. We all have a *lot* to learn about sex, and acknowledging your own limitations while expressing a willingness to learn and adapt will set the tone for your partner to do the same—at his or her own pace. Sex is the one activity that we engage in without any structured education or observation, so we *need* direction. Start the conversation with a few inquiries:

"Do you like when I . . . ?"

"Show me how you like it . . ."

"In an ideal world, how many times per week/ month would you want to have sex?"

"After you climax, how do you want to be touched/held?"

"If I were to seduce you tomorrow, what would you want me to do?"

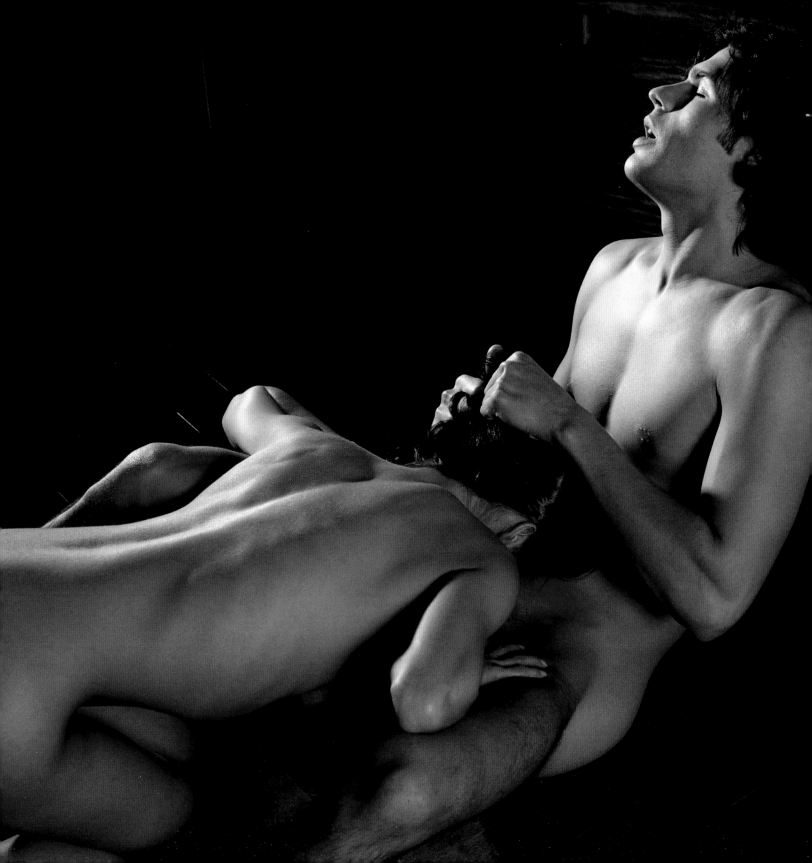

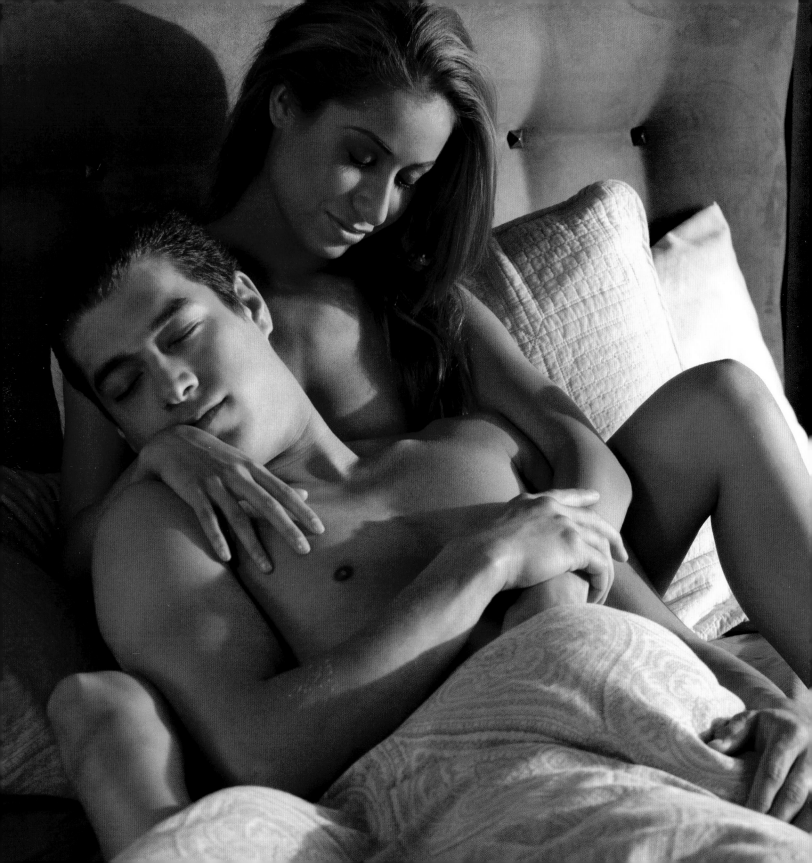

EXPRESS DESIRES WITH CARE

As you become accustomed to highlighting the positive and asking questions, your comfort level with talking about sex will increase and you'll likely find yourself making requests and setting boundaries with greater ease. Expressing your desires and interests with care and tact can be a challenge. Assertion skills are best learned in low-stress situations, and sex doesn't usually qualify as such. Learning to ask for what you want in other realms *outside* of the bedroom is one of the most effective ways to develop strong sexual communication skills. It may be difficult at first, but being honest about your boundaries and needs can be empowering, and with time these communication skills will begin to arise naturally, translating into greater satisfaction in the bedroom. You may want to encourage your lover to share her requests first so that you can model receptiveness to her needs.

When revealing new desires and fantasies, bear in mind that sensitivity is of paramount importance. You are already aware of your lover's insecurities and soft spots, so work around them with grace as much as possible. If you're met with discomfort, jealousy, or indications of insecurity, be as supportive as possible by listening and offering reassurance. We often respond to negative emotions with more negative emotions instead of looking for the source of the problem. Making an effort to see things from your partner's perspective can make awkward conversations less stressful and more productive.

Consider trying these conversation starters when making sexual requests:

"I would love more_____. You're so good at it."

"I had a dream about trying _____ with you and it got me thinking…"

"I read an article about_____. What do you think of that?"

"I have the best orgasms when you _____."

"In an ideal world, I'd like to have sex (however you define it) X times per week. What can we do to make more time/find a balance?"

"One thing I'd like to work on is…"

Talking about sex isn't a one-shot deal. It's an ongoing conversation that can include laughter, tension, and awkward moments. It is that tension and awkwardness that will only intensify passion and attraction later on. So relax, take a deep breath, and start talking! You'll be glad you did.

HOTTER ORAL: DIRTY TALK

Dirty talk is the skill that all good lovers have in common. Once you learn to talk your lover's ear off in bed, you'll barely need to move a muscle—other than your tongue, of course. This is because dirty talk allows you to bring his hottest fantasies to life in words. Through dirty talk, your nasty little tongue becomes the conduit that bridges his deepest desires with in-the-flesh sex. And since fantasy is almost always hotter than reality, fulfilling his desires through dirty talk can be hotter than the real thing. So get ready to whisper sweet (or not-so-sweet) nothings in his ear and watch the fireworks unfold!

Many people find dirty talk off-putting or embarrassing because they derive their definitions and expectations from porn. This leaves them with a terribly limited repertoire that often excludes the highly personal element of individual fantasy. The content of mainstream porn also suggests that all dirty talk must be raunchy, hard core, and deeply rooted in gendered stereotypes of sexual experience. In reality, nothing could be further from the truth. Dirty talk does not need to be rough, naughty, or even sexual to be erotic. The most enticing chatter can be romantic, teasing, alluring, and flirtatious according to your personal preferences.

If you're new to talking dirty, begin with some generous but honest verbal feedback that includes moans, groans, deep exhales, or other sounds to let your lover know that you're enjoying yourself. Don't feel the need to exaggerate—sexy talk is even hotter when you let the tension mount gradually.

Start Small

When you're ready, toss in a few words and short phrases ranging from "Yes!," "More!," and "Ahhh" to "Whoa!," "Wow," and "Fuck yeah!" Use language that comes naturally to you, as opposed to repeating what you have seen in films or read online. And since dirty talk goes both ways, use a few simple lines to develop greater comfort as you explore your lover's body: "Do you like that?" "Where do you want it?" "What can I do for you?" "Tell me how you like it." "Lie back and let me give it to you."

Indulge Your Sense of Humor

As you integrate dirty talk into your sexual repertoire, remember that it is okay to giggle a little. Obviously you don't want to laugh *at* your lover, but having a healthy sense of humor will help to ease the tension when you are experimenting with new language, tone, and subject matter. In fact, using a bit of humor and playfulness may be the ideal approach if talking dirty makes you blush or if you're worried about how your lover will respond.

Set Ground Rules

If you are going to continue to expand your dirty talk repertoire, chat with your partner ahead of time about topics, fantasies, or words that are off-limits. Each person has her own unique set of limitations and sensitivities. Maybe your partner likes to use the word *pussy,* but it makes you angry—not a good mood to be in in the sack! Since these sensitivities can change over time, it's a good idea to revisit your ground rules periodically.

Remember that sex talk isn't enjoyable to all people, especially those who have survived a sexual hardship. As Dr. Ruth Neustifter (aka Dr. Ruthie) notes, "The purpose of talking dirty is to help you both feel excited and intimate, not to feel awkward or triggered! Explicit language can be fun, but it's not erotic for everyone and that's okay."

Experiment with Variety

Dirty talk comes in many forms, so experiment with a variety of styles to find the ones that suit you both best. Whether you prefer to be romantic, alluring, teasing, aggressive, demanding, responsive, descriptive, naughty, instructive, ego-stroking, or fantastical is entirely up to you!

Play with these lines on your own in front of the mirror or while masturbating as you get comfortable with your own personal style:

DR. JESS SAYS . . .

Be honest with regard to your fantasies and remember that sexual fantasies may be at odds with your desired reality. Just because *talking* about attending a sex party gets you all riled up in the heat of the moment does not mean that you need to pursue this fantasy in real life. It is important to set boundaries before sex play and debrief after sex to discuss how you feel about the things that were said.

FOR SEX GEEKS

Communication outside of the bedroom isn't the only form of dialogue that lays the groundwork for a hot sex life. Research shows that talking about sex *during* sex leads to higher levels of sexual satisfaction. A study conducted by researchers at Cleveland State University in Ohio found that those who communicate during sex have higher levels of sexual self-esteem and satisfaction. But if dirty talk still isn't on your sexual radar, the same study found that nonverbal communication cues also boost sexual enjoyment.

STYLES OF DIRTY TALK

ROMANTIC
"You're the only one for me!"
"I'll only ever want you."
"You're everything I've ever dreamed of."
"You're my dream guy/girl."

ALLURING
"I know you want what's under this shirt."
"Tell me what you'd do to me."
"Make my thighs wet!"
"I'll do whatever you tell me to do."

TEASING
"You can't have me."
"If you want it, come and get it."
"Pour me a glass of wine and I'll think about it . . ."
"You know you want it."

AGGRESSIVE
"I'm going to hold you down and make you come."
"Behave or I'll give you something to scream about."
"Do as you're told if you want a piece of me."
"Take it!"

DEMANDING
"Lay me down and take care of me now!"
"Get down on your knees and do it how I like it."
"I want it in my mouth."
"Suck it."

RESPONSIVE
"Tell me how you like it."
"What can I do for you?"
"I'm just going to lie back and let you work me over."
"It feels so good."

DESCRIPTIVE
"I'm going to make you scream."
"I'm coming!"
"I can see your hot body in the mirror."
"It feels so good."

NAUGHTY
"I want to taste your hot cum."
"I thought about you last night when I was touching myself."
"Tie me down and have your way with me."
"I want to be your hot slut."

INSTRUCTIVE
"Put your hand right here!"
"Nibble on me a little."
"Don't stop!"
"Put in your mouth."

EGO-STROKING
"You're the best I've ever had."
"You make me so wet/horny/excited."
"You taste like honey."
"I would pay for this!"

FANTASTICAL
"I want to watch you with another man."
"Let's have a little threesome and let her taste your big cock."
"I want to be tied up and spanked until I can't take it anymore."
"Tie me down and force it down my throat."

ORAL SEX MOVES SHE'LL LOVE

Whether you're using your tongue, your lips, or your fingers, these moves will have her screaming your name. Remember that variety is key and you can adjust (and even rename) each of these techniques to make them your own. If you just can't wait to try them all, remember that you already know what she likes, so add new techniques into the mix one or two at a time.

It is not uncommon for women (and men) to feel uncomfortable with their bodies during oral sex, but you can help to put her at ease by expressing your thoughts and desires with honesty and effusion. If you love going down on her, be sure to let her know with your sounds, words, breath, facial expressions, and body language. Her pleasure is as much related to your attitude and enjoyment as it is to the techniques you employ, so let your enthusiasm shine.

THE ROCKET

The Rocket is one of the most versatile finger and tongue tricks designed to make her toes curl at any stage of the sexual response cycle. Whether you want to seduce her into your arms or bring her to the heights of an earth-shattering orgasm, this will become a go-to move for years to come.

Take Position

You can use the Rocket technique in almost any position. Whether you're sitting side-by-side at dinner or lying on the couch watching a movie, as long as you can cup her mons into your hand and reach your fingers down against her lips, you're ready to go!

The Moves

Place your palm flat against her mons and bend your fingers down to press against the full width and length of her vulva so that you're cupping it in your hand.

Slowly slide your fingers up and down ever so slightly, maintaining pressure against her mons and clitoris.

If you're able, continue to slide your fingers up and down as you slip your tongue between the grooves of your fingers to tease her inner lips.

Increase the pressure and speed of your fingers, paying special attention to the very top of her vulva as she becomes more aroused.

SIT ON MY FACE

This oral sex move allows her to maintain complete control as she directs the pressure, depth, speed, and motion with her hips. Her directives not only ensure that she gets it exactly as she pleases, but her dominance offers great practice in sexual assertion.

If you love the Sit on My Face technique but want to keep things fresh, simply change directions to face his feet and ask him to finger your bum a little at the same time.

Take Position
Lie on your back and prop your head up with a few pillows. Have her kneel over your lower face with her back to your feet so that you can use eye contact as a means of communicating while your mouth is full.

The Moves
How she sits on your face is entirely up to her, but here are a few suggestions for her:

Rock your hips back and forth in an elliptical fashion.

Demand that he stick his tongue straight up as you pop up and down over it.

Apply some lube and slide back and forth over the full length of his face.

Rub your wet pussy against his chin and closed lips with firm pressure.

Sway your hips from side to side in a semi-circle.

Sit hard on his mouth and instruct him to suck away.

Ask him to stick his tongue out flat against his chin and grind up on it.

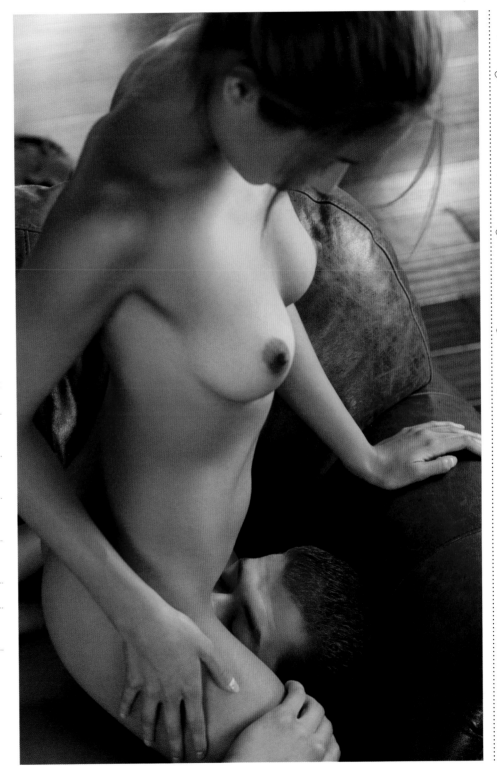

SEX TIPS FROM
THE PROS

Slide three wet fingers beneath your mouth
and stroke her sweet spot (perineum) from
back to front in rhythm with your tongue
twirling.

SWEET SUCTION

This technique not only combines licking,
sucking, and deep pressure, but it also provides
full-contact stimulation of the entire vulva.
By wrapping your mouth all the way around
the outer edges of her pussy, you'll titillate and
awaken all the inner and outer components of her
highly responsive clitoris.

Take Position
Kneel on a pillow on the floor next to the bed
as she lies down with her knees bent and legs
hanging off the edge.

The Moves

Tease all around her pussy with some gentle
breath kisses without allowing your lips to
contact her skin. Breathe heavily over her thighs
and mons, allowing your cheeks and nose to
touch her only incidentally.

With a wide, flat tongue lick from the very
bottom of her vulva up to the top as slowly as
possible. Repeat this lick in the same direction for
thirty to sixty seconds.

Switch directions and lick from her clitoral
glans down to her fourchette (where her inner
labia meet at the bottom) using the warm, flat
underside of your tongue. Repeat for another
minute.

When she starts to thrust her hips into you, open
your mouth wide and press your lips around the
outer edges of her vulva.

Sweep your tongue around the inside perimeter
of your lips while sucking and slurping away.

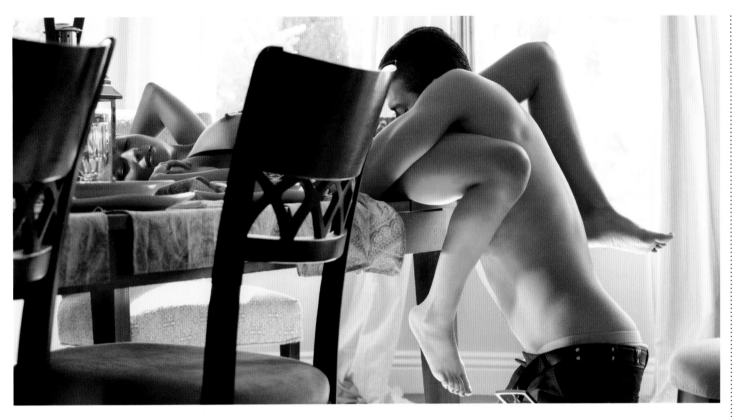

LOLLIPOPS

If you want to spread her orgasmic sensations across the entire surface of her pussy and beyond, then the Lollipops move is right up your alley. Using sweeping motions to stroke the bulbs of her inner clitoris from the top of her clitoral glans to her fourchette down below, this move provides the intense stimulation most women require to reach the heights of sexual pleasure.

Take Position
Kneel between her legs as she sits (or lies) atop a table with her legs hanging off the edge.

The Moves

Warm her up with a gentle thigh massage by circling with only the palms of your hands slathered in coconut oil.

As her body begins to relax into your hands, slide one palm up to her mons and press down gently as the other flat palm circles slowly around her entire vulva.

Lick her pussy like a lollipop with a soft flat tongue, starting from the fourchette at the very bottom all the way up to the clitoral glans at the top. Alternate from the "left lane" of her vulva to the "right lane" as you separate her lips with your tongue with each stroke.

Between each lick, wrap your lips around the tiny fourchette at the base as you suck gently. Then press your tongue firmly into her clit at the top.

SEX TIPS FROM THE PROS

Twirl your tongue around her fourchette and then lick with a wide, flat tongue up to her clit before encircling it with the tip of your tongue.

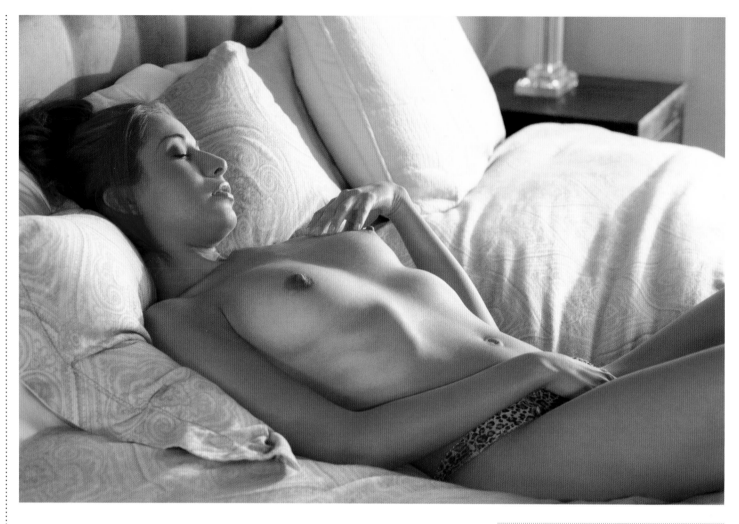

STROKING THE SHAFT

For many women, the shaft of the clitoris offers an immense sense of pleasure, and, just like men, orgasm is often the result of a rhythmic stroking motion. Slide your smooth fingers over this hot spot while simultaneously kissing and rubbing her inner clitoral legs and bulbs to send her into sensory overload.

Take Position

Prop up her hips and lower back with at least two pillows and spread her legs wide as she bends her knees. Slide between her open legs and dive on in!

The Moves

Press your full lips against her vulva and slide them up and down.

Move your entire head in a circular fashion to encircle her entire pussy with your wet lips.

Pulse your lips against her as you slide your tongue inside and curl it up against her soft, inner walls.

Add your fingers into the mix according to your preferences as you increase the pace, depth, and intensity of your tongue screw.

As her arousal levels rise, press your tongue flat against her vulva and stroke from side to side.

Continue to shake your head from side to side with your tongue pressed into her and place one thumb on her clitoral hood. Draw her skin up and down with your thumb to stroke the shaft and produce a climactic finale.

SUCK ME IN

Primal thrusting makes oral sex play even hotter, and the Suck Me In move allows you to pull her into your face in the most carnal of ways. The sensation of being tongue-screwed, coupled with the intimacy of your kiss, creates the perfect combination to take her over the edge.

Take Position

Kneel on the floor next to the bed between her legs as they dangle off the edge or rest on your shoulders. She can lie back and enjoy being serviced, reach down and lend a hand to a good cause, or grab you by the hair to intensify and control your thrusting.

The Moves

Slide your hands beneath her butt cheeks and hold her in place while you breathe warm air between her legs.

Breathe in deeply and tell her how much you love it.

Roll the sides of your tongue together into a tube and slide it inside of her while you press your lips into her to create wet suction. If you can't hold your tongue in a tube on its own, you can still perform this sensational move.

As her breathing increases and she begins to moan, squeeze her butt cheeks into your palms and draw her into your face.

Pick up the pace of the tongue screwing and lip suction as you thrust her pussy in and out with salacious delight.

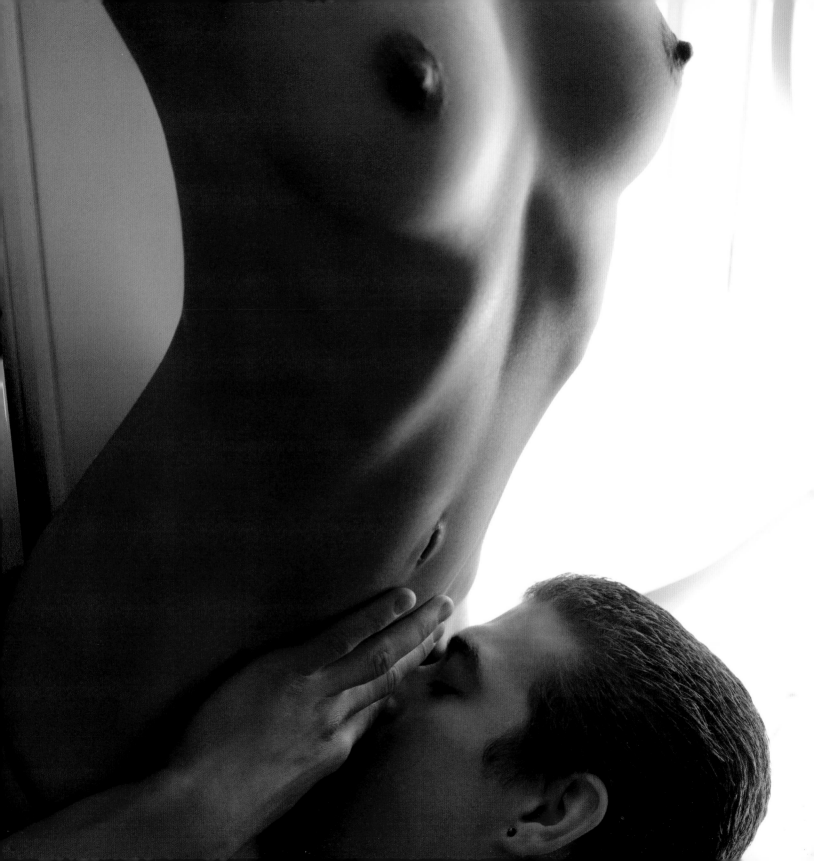

G-SPOT GUSHER

Get her wet and let her gush as you excite her G-spot from all angles and leave her dripping at the thighs.

Alternate the "come hither" motion against her G-spot with some deep circular pressure. Draw circles or ovals on the upper vaginal wall, against the G-spot. You should feel the area swell as circulation and arousal rise.

Remember that the G-spot isn't a distinct organ but an area of the body that is associated with the release of fluids. Each woman's experience with the G-spot is unique, and the degree of pleasure associated with this sensitive area can vary according to a number of factors, including arousal levels and monthly cycle.

Take Position

Kneel at her feet as she stands with her back against a wall.

The Moves

Play with your surefire warm-up moves that you know she loves *before* moving on to her sensitive G-spot.

Once she's all fired up and ready to go, slide your index and middle fingers inside of her and curl them up against the front wall of her vagina (toward her stomach). Curl them in a "come hither" motion, gradually increasing the pressure and speed, up to at least two "curls" per second.

As you curl your fingers inside of her, wrap your lips around the glans of her clit and pulse in tempo with your fingers.

Finally, press your lower palm down against her lower abdomen to squeeze and excite her prostate from the inside-out.

SEX TIP FROM THE PROS

Though squirting (page 136) isn't a sideshow trick, and not every woman will experience the same degree of ejaculation, you can encourage fluid expulsion by bearing down with your pelvic floor muscles. As you approach orgasm, take a few deep breaths as you "push out" with the muscles around your vagina.

FACE LIFT

Many women reach the heights of orgasm through heavy pressure and friction against the outer parts of their nether regions. The Face Lift technique uses the weight of her body along with vibrations and pressure from below to take her over the edge.

Don't be afraid to get your entire face in there. In fact, you can slide the tip of your nose right inside of her and circle it around the sensitive opening of her vagina.

Take Position
Lie on your back and have her lie on top of you facedown—either facing your feet or your head—with her pussy in your face. If it's more comfortable, she can also kneel over your face.

The Moves

Reach around and grab her butt cheeks with both hands as you pull her into your face.

Shake your head from side-to-side as though you're saying "No!" and moan a little so she feels the vibrations against her clit.

Alternate between nodding "Yes" and shaking your head "No" and continue to breathe deeply.

Talk with your mouth full and tell her just how much you love it:

"You taste so good."

"I can't get enough. Mmm."

"I want to swallow your cum."

"Your pussy is so beautiful and sweet."

Wrap your mouth around her entire pussy (the outer parts of it) and suck ravenously as you taste her juices.

Slide your hands onto her hips to guide her in setting the pace. As she thrusts into your mouth, lift your face to increase the friction and pressure. Hold on to her so that as you force her hips into the air with your face, you maintain constant contact and connection.

Take her to the next level by adding a vibrator into the mix. Hold it firmly between your lips (with a little extra support from your hands for safety) as she lowers herself onto it and really gets into the groove of "screwing" your face.

TONGUE SCREW

As your nimble fingers press into her G-spot and squeeze her clitoris, your tongue works its magic against her responsive lower wall, resulting in a climactic flurry of nerve-ending responses.

Take Position
Kneel behind her as she lies flat on her stomach with her legs hanging off the bed and her feet on the floor. Approaching from behind will facilitate the dual entry of your fingers in alignment with your tongue.

The Moves

Sweep your fingers gently over her butt cheeks and tease her perineum as you breathe over her pussy from behind.

With your palm facing downward, slide your index finger inside of her and slip your thumb beneath her.

Gently pinch your thumb and index finger together so that your thumb presses against her clit and your index finger curls against her G-spot along the front wall.

Angle your other knuckles downward to make space for your tongue. Slide your tongue inside of her against your index finger and curl upward (toward the back wall of her vagina) as you continue the pinching motion.

SLIPPERY PALM

The Slippery Palm technique puts you in the driver's seat as you use your strong hands to hold her open and leave her feeling vulnerable to your sexual prowess. Her most sensitive areas will be exposed, so encourage her to embrace the submissive role as you work your magic between her legs.

Take Position

Sweep her off of her feet and place her on the bed. Reassure her that she's in good hands. Lie on a pillow between her legs as she rests her feet (legs bent) on your shoulders. Place a few pillows under her hips for easy access as she lies on her back.

The Moves

Tie a blindfold loosely around her eyes.

S-l-o-w-l-y kiss your way down from her neck to her inner thighs, stopping to show some love to her collarbone, nipples, underarms, hips bones, and bellybutton along the way.

Slip both palms in between her legs and warm up her thighs with soft, circular strokes as you kiss her mons with wet lips and a swirling tongue.

Press your palms into her vulva and use your thumbs to separate her inner lips and reveal the shiny space between them.

Sweep your tongue around this opening while you press your thumbs gently against her inner lips and slide them ever-so-slightly up and down.

Use the textured upper side of your tongue to trace a large X over her exposed area and moan a little to let her know you're enjoying yourself.

If she seems tense or tries to close her legs at all, scold her gently: "You're all mine and I'm going to take care of you, so you best behave."

Open your mouth wide and press your lips and flat tongue against her vestibule as you slide from top to bottom while sucking away.

FAQ: IT DOESN'T FEEL GOOD WHEN MY HUSBAND GOES DOWN ON ME. HOW DO I TEACH HIM WHAT I LIKE WITHOUT HURTING HIS FEELINGS?

Dr. Ruthie offers the following advice: "You're in the perfect place by having this book in your hand; now try sharing it with your husband! When you read a tip in this book that you like, suggest the two of you playfully experiment with it, and encourage him to suggest new moves, too. When he makes a motion during oral sex that you enjoy, stop and point it out with excitement then ask him to do more of it (faster, higher, harder, or however you need it). Most lovers really want to please, so helping them repeat and expand on their best moves is a great motivator. Eventually the things that aren't praised are likely to vanish from the menu. He is also likely to enjoy hearing you describe how his best moves feel to you—and want to hear more!"

SEX TIPS FROM THE PROS

Practice this one on your finger to familiarize yourself with the sensation of suction created by a cradled tongue. You should almost be able to hold your finger in place with the sides of your tongue as they curl up around your finger.

THE HOTTEST MOVES FOR HIM

Though you may already be well versed in the art of oral sex, even the most talented temptress can use a refresher from time to time. These tongue and finger techniques are designed for the woman who wants to spoil him with heavenly pleasure . . . and of course reap her own rewards.

TONGUE CRADLE

Engulf his entire girth between your lips and tongue to create a cradle that's warm, wet, and brimming with suction. As your tongue envelops the sensitive underside of his cock (including the inner spongy tissue and the sensitive notch known as the frenulum), your tight lips wrap around the swollen ridge to send him over the edge and keep him coming back for more!

Take Position
Let him sit back and relax in his favorite armchair as you kneel on a pillow at his feet. Depending on the chair height, your heights, and the angle of his erection, you can add pillows to avoid straining your neck.

The Moves

Work him up with some shallow sucks, swallows, and strokes, and move on to the Tongue Cradle when you feel his cock swelling and his balls tightening upward.

Wrap your lips around his shaft and press your tongue into the underside, allowing the sides of your tongue to curl upward to wrap around the sides of his cock. Stick your tongue out just enough to cover your lower lip so that you form a tight cradle between your upper lip and your tongue.

Suck greedily on the upper half of his cock, pressing your tongue firmly into him to feel the sensitive notch of connective tissue just below his head (on the underside) and tightening your grip with your lip as you slide over his swollen ridge.

Increase the suction and pace to stroke up and down every half second until you feel his cock pulsing in your mouth.

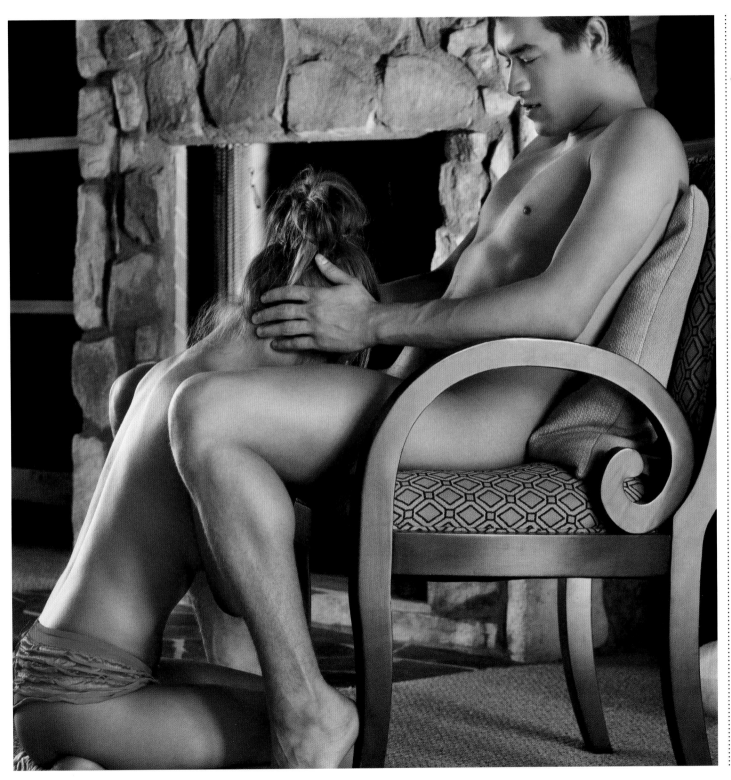

ALL YOUR LOVE

Look up at him while performing the All Your Love technique so that you see his eyes roll back into his head! As your warm, wet hands encircle his sensitive lower shaft, your tight lips titillate his innervated upper half to send him into a fit of delight.

Take Position

Lie on your back as he bends over you on his hands and knees to dip his cock into your mouth. He will have to lower his butt slightly, or you can prop your head up with a pillow.

The Moves

Begin with your hands against his lower abs so that you can control how deep he thrusts. Suck his head into your mouth and twirl your tongue all the way around his swollen ridge.

Spend a few minutes sucking only on his head before adding some lube and wrapping both hands around his base, one on top of the other.

Lower your lips halfway down his shaft to meet your fingers and increase your speed and suction as you stroke with your hands in rhythm with your mouth.

Alternate between stroking with two hands and sucking with your mouth according to what feels best for you.

As his arousal increases, wrap both wet hands around his shaft and twist in opposite directions as though you are wringing out a wet towel. At the same time, suck on his head and upper shaft with a warm, tight mouth, twisting as you pass over his swollen ridge.

As you twist your hands from side to side, be sure to stroke up and down to draw his hot come out into your mouth.

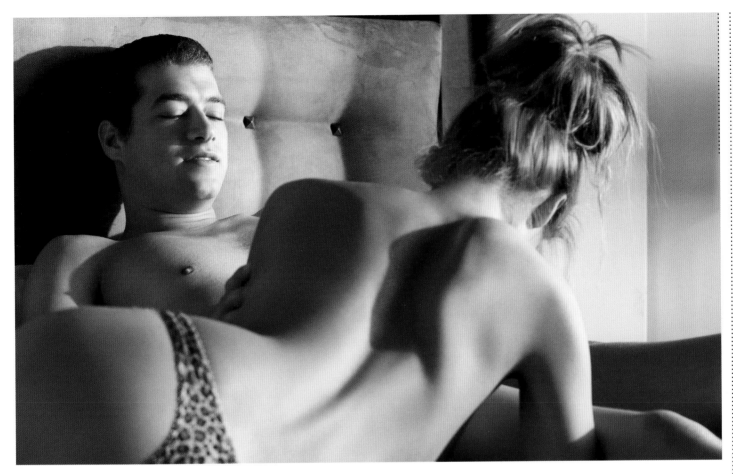

TWIST AND SHOUT

Wrap your lips around his most responsive spot, the frenulum, and watch him moan and melt like putty in your hands . . . and mouth. A simple quarter turn at the top of his shaft coupled with some tongue action against his frenulum makes the Twist and Shout a top-rated finishing move.

Take Position

Kneel at his side as he sits back against the headboard. Approaching from the side is essential to this move, and it will be easier on your neck if he's sitting at an angle that allows his erection to point toward the ceiling.

The Moves

Start with his favorite moves to tease his cock to attention.

Wrap your lips around his shaft at the deepest point possible and suck upward. When you reach the area just below the coronal ridge, twist your mouth around his head and flick your tongue powerfully against his frenulum.

Slide back down to the base by turning your head back to your starting position, facing him from the side.

Repeat this subtle twist at the top as you suck away at a rhythmic pace.

DR. JESS SAYS . . .

If you have difficulty with the Twist and Shout, try it using your hands. Simply slather them in lube, stroke up to the top, and perform a tiny twist and you increase the pressure at the very top of the shaft below the head.

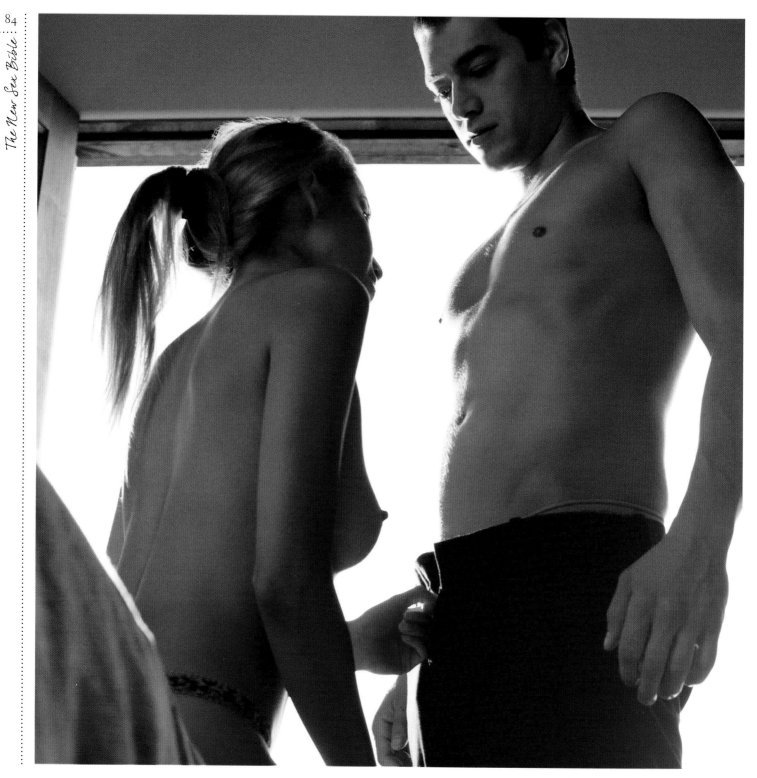

BETTER THAN DEEP THROAT

Thanks to the magic and special effects of porn, "deep throating" has been elevated to a level of fame and reverence beyond its true merits. Though deep pressure, suction, and stroking are certainly desirable, they're not the be-all, end-all of a good blow job. After all, your hands offer not only a tighter grip and greater flexibility, but with the right amount of lube and perfected technique, they should feel wetter and better than your mouth alone.

Take Position

Lie on your back with your head hanging off the bed to ensure that your throat is elongated. Have him stand on the floor facing you as he presses his cock against your eager cheeks. He can opt to be selfish and revel in your sensual skills (everyone enjoys a turn at being a taker once in a while), or he can play with your hair and fondle your breasts while enjoying the sexy view from above.

The Moves

Warm your hands up in advance (using warm water, if necessary) so they reach a temperature similar to that of your mouth.

Interlace your fingers as you clasp both hands together and slather them in lube. (If using two hands is difficult to execute, then try this with one.)

Attach your interlaced hands to your mouth so they become one fluid unit.

Breathe heavily so that it feels as though you're approaching him with your warm, wet mouth and slide your hands and mouth over his cock in one fell swoop.

Lower your hands all the way to his base and then tighten your grip as you suck right back up to the top.

Stroke and suck up and down with your hands and mouth as one long, wet tunnel, squeezing a little tighter each time you reach the very base.

FAQ: HOW IMPORTANT IS IT TO SWALLOW HIS COME?

Swallowing is a matter of personal taste. Some men love it and others are relatively indifferent. Similarly, some women love the taste of come and others find it rather unappealing. If you're a bit reticent to swallow, start with a little at a time. He can spray the rest on your breasts or stomach. Swallowing is just one of an infinite number of potentially sexy acts, so don't feel any pressure to perform either way.

THE REAL DEAL

When it comes to mind-blowing oral, sometimes it's what's on the inside that counts! Not only does your attitude, enthusiasm, and enjoyment make for the most exceptional experience, but paying attention to the *inner penis* may just be what it takes to make him scream your name. Stroke and suck all the way down to the oft-neglected bulb of his penis and he won't know what hit him!

Take Position

You'll need easy access to the perineum (that fleshy part behind his balls) for this one, so try the Real Deal on your knees as he stands against the wall in the shower or behind the blinds of his office. Surprise!

The Moves

Suck him into your mouth, squeezing tightly as you suck upward and releasing slightly as you stroke downward with your lips.

Add your tongue into the mix, allowing it to wrap sensually around the midsection of his shaft.

Grab him by the hips to encourage him to set the pace with a little thrusting, and let your natural sounds emanate as they arise.

Rub some lube on one hand and reach behind his balls toward his bum. Place all four fingers against his taint and press deeply.

Stroke forward with all four fingers toward his balls as you suck upward from the base and stroke back toward his pucker (butt hole) as you lower your lips back down to form a fluid motion between your lips and fingers.

Increase your speed and squeeze even tighter with your wet lips as you press deeper into his perineum with your fingers.

When he's ready to come slide your fingers back toward his butt and pulse firmly against him just in front of his pucker.

FAQ: WHAT SHOULD I DO WHEN HE'S COMING?

That's a great question, and the only person who can answer it is him. Men seem to be split on type of stimulation, pressure, and speed they enjoy during orgasm, so you'll have to do a bit of prying. If you're reading this book, you can use this chapter as the perfect opportunity to ask him.

Dr. Jess insists!

Another way to find out what he likes is to watch him finish himself off. Ask him to come all over your breasts and take mental notes on his technique. Does he stroke the full length or avoid the head? Does he slow down his pace or keep it up? And when he's finished, does he hold on with all his might or release completely?

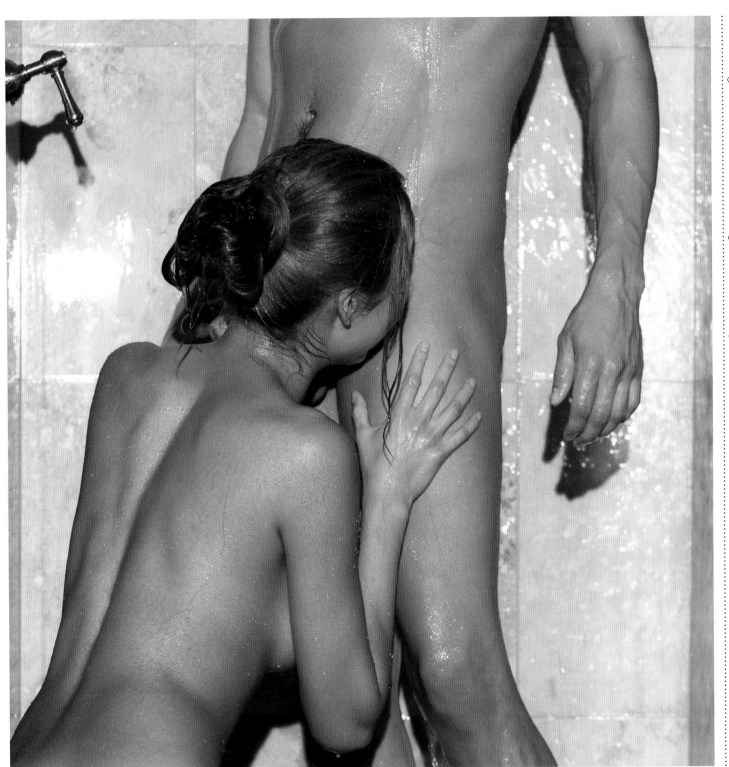

WETTER, TIGHTER, BETTER

This intimate blow job technique offers the tightest squeeze possible as you clench his manhood between your teeth. But before you both start squirming, rest assured that the warm padding of your upper lip and tongue protect him from your sharp cuspids and make this move a sure-fire favorite.

Take Position

This highly versatile move can be performed in almost any position from any angle. Be sure to use lube because your upper lip does not provide natural lubrication.

The Moves

Cover your lower teeth with your tongue by sticking it out ever-so-slightly and wrap your upper lip over your upper row of teeth. This should create a tight pocket between your tongue and teeth that can provide lots of pressure against his cock.

Apply a generous portion of lube and slide your lips and tongue over him, clamping down as you suck. When you reach the deepest point, bite/clamp a bit harder, drawing upward with all your might.

FAQ: WHAT LUBE SHOULD I USE FOR ORAL SEX?

Flavored lubes come in both water- and silicone-based formulas, and several brands now offer glycerin- and paraben-free versions. Sliquid Swirl Green Apple is sweetened with aspartame, and Hathor Aphrodisia's Lubricant Lickeurs use the natural botanical sweetener stevia. If you prefer an unflavored lube, try water-based Blossom Organics or silicone-based Uberlube. Better yet, pay a visit your local sex store and do some live taste testing before you buy!

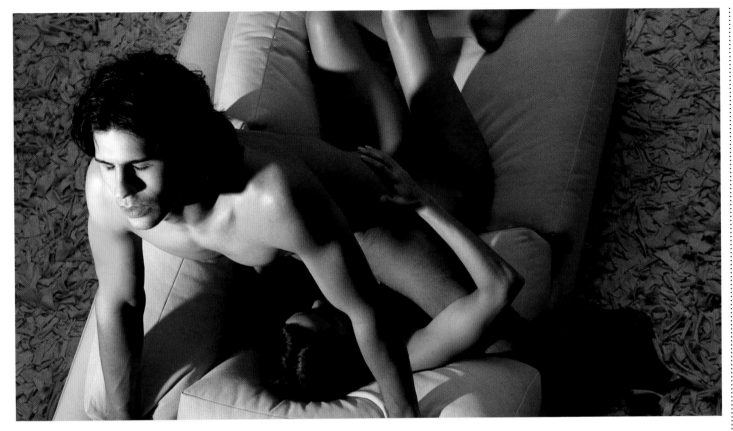

SWEET SWALLOW

Use the powerful muscles of your mouth and throat to pulse and tighten against his bulging head as you suck him in.

Take Position

Lie on your sides facing one another and work your way down to between his legs.

The Moves

Tease him a little as you press your cheeks into his shaft, or smack his cock gently against your face.

Flick your tongue against the tip of his cock, licking away any pre-come and swallowing hard.

Slide your lips over his head and wrap them around the top of his shaft below the ridge and swallow deeply.

Look him in the eye and tell him you want to taste him.

Suck in your usual fashion until his cock swells with excitement, and then lower your lips to the base or to your deepest level of comfort.

Once you reach your greatest depth, swallow as deeply as possible, constricting your throat around the head of his cock. Repeat these swallowing motions every second as you allow the saliva to drip out of your mouth.

If the deep swallows make you feel uncomfortable, you can also use your lips and tongue to create the swallowing sensation around his head and shaft.

FAQ: WHAT IS PRE-COME?

Pre-come, or pre-ejaculatory fluid, is an alkaline substance released during sexual arousal. Released by the Cowper's glands, this small amount of clear fluid prepares the urethra for the protected passage of sperm by neutralizing it acidity. Though pre-come does not contain sperm, it can transport "leftover" swimmers that remain in the urethra from a previous ejaculation; peeing after you ejaculate can clear the urethra of residual sperm, but it does *not* prevent the transmission of sexually transmitted infections.

DR. JESS SAYS . . .

Since the Screw involves power play between dominant and submissive roles, you'll need to pre-select a safe signal that indicates cease and desist. Two taps to the back of his thigh or a snap of your fingers should suffice, but be sure to agree upon this signal with clarity ahead of time.

THE SCREW

This technique requires a good amount of trust and the ability to communicate using nonverbal cues. By shifting the reins of control over to the man, the Screw ensures that he gets everything he wants as he sets the depth, speed, motion, and tone of the encounter. See note left.

Take Position

Drop to your knees at his feet as he stands over you against a wall.

The Moves for Her

Place his hands on the back of your head and look up at him. Tell him your soft lips, strong tongue, and warm mouth are all his and let him guide you with his hands.

If at any point you feel uncomfortable, tap him twice on the back of his thigh to signal that you need to stop.

The Moves for Him

Use your hands to gradually guide her lips over your cock.

Press her face into your groin as deeply as you want it and pull her hair to make her slide back up to the tip.

Place your hands on her cheeks and rotate gently if you like circular motions. Give her direct instructions to ensure you're fully satisfied:

"More tongue."

"Suck harder."

"Slow down."

"Lick your lips."

"Open your eyes and look up at me."

Pay attention to her hands to take note of your safe signal.

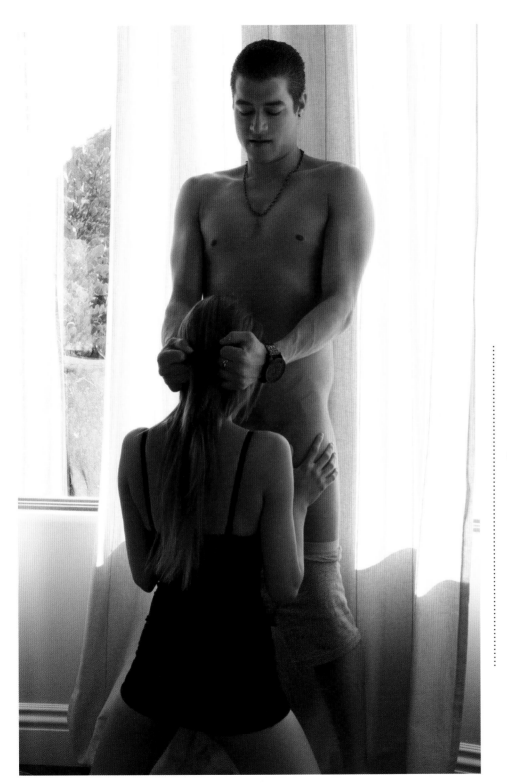

FAQ: HOW DO I TAKE HIM IN DEEPER DURING ORAL SEX?

Lady Kay, a high-end escort, offers this advice: "Deep throating is a skill that took me some time to perfect. It seems to come easier when I'm both relaxed and turned on, and I usually have to try different angles, depending on the curve of his penis. To ease into it, I breathe slowly through my nose, inhaling as I suck him in and exhaling as he pulls out. If I'm enjoying it, my mouth gets wetter, and I let the saliva run out of my mouth so that it doesn't tickle my throat. Sometimes I'll suck him in deeper by yawning, because this seems to minimize my gag reflex. If I do start to gag, I just exaggerate my inhalations to ward off the reflex."

THE TEMPLE

Create a long, tight tunnel of suction and twist all around his most sensitive areas to introduce him to a sexual ecstasy beyond his wildest dreams.

Take Position

As he lies on his back, kneel over his chest facing his feet. You're going to have your bum fairly far back, almost as if you're in the 69 position.

The Moves

Bend over and rub his cock between your well-lubed palms in sweeping circular motions as you breathe over his balls.

Get your tongue in on the action by licking broad strokes between your sweeping palms.

Place your hands in prayer position, apply a generous serving of lube, and attach them to your lips thumbs-first to create an elongated version of your mouth.

Lower over his cock pinky-first as you suck him into your wet, tight palms and mouth. Stroke from tip to base building speed, tension, and suction as you slide up and down.

Add some tight pulses at the base and twirl around subtly as you reach the midsection of his shaft with your fingers. Your tight hands will grip his shaft as your lips pass over his frenulum.

Pick up the pace and moan enthusiastically to convey your pleasure and allow him to feel the vibrations against his cock.

SEX TIPS FROM THE PROS

Emily Muse from Muse Massage Spa says, "Mind his balls! Use them to control his orgasm. Hold them close to help him cum. Tug them lightly to delay his orgasm."

TWO THUMBS UP

This technique requires some coordination, but a few minutes of practice will be well worth the orgasmic rewards. Using both your hands and mouth, the Two Thumbs Up allows you to activate nerve endings in three of his most excitable hot spots: his balls, the lower third of his shaft, and the underside of his head.

Take Position

Positioning is important, as you need to be able to tuck your head between his legs in order to suck his balls right into your mouth. Try this one on your knees as he relaxes in his favorite armchair or let him sit on the edge of the (sturdy) kitchen table.

The Moves

Climb between his legs and sweep your tongue lightly around the edge of his balls. Trace a figure-eight shape over the front and scoop your tongue underneath to lick the responsive rear surface.

As you twirl your tongue around, slather your hands in lube and clasp the base of his cock with one hand as lightly as possible. Stroke up to the top holding his cock with one hand as loosely as possible to pique his interest. Alternate hands for several strokes ensuring that your touch is featherlight.

After a minute or two, increase the pressure of your strokes and wrap two hands around his base, interlacing your fingers with your thumbs pointing straight up toward the tip. Add lube to ensure it's super slippery.

Stroke upward and sweep the pads of your thumbs in a circular or heart-shaped motion when you reach his frenulum, the soft skin on the underside of his head. Increase the pressure as you squeeze both hands around the lower third of his shaft and suck his balls right into your mouth.

Coordinate twirling your tongue around his balls or sucking downward on them as you stroke upward and massage his frenulum and head to elongate his full unit. As you squeeze around his lower shaft, gently press his balls up toward his body with your lips.

DR. JESS SAYS . . .

The Two Thumbs Up move may sound technical, but you don't have to follow the instructions to a T. There is no universally right or wrong way to perform oral sex, so use these guidelines as inspiration as opposed to a perfect recipe.

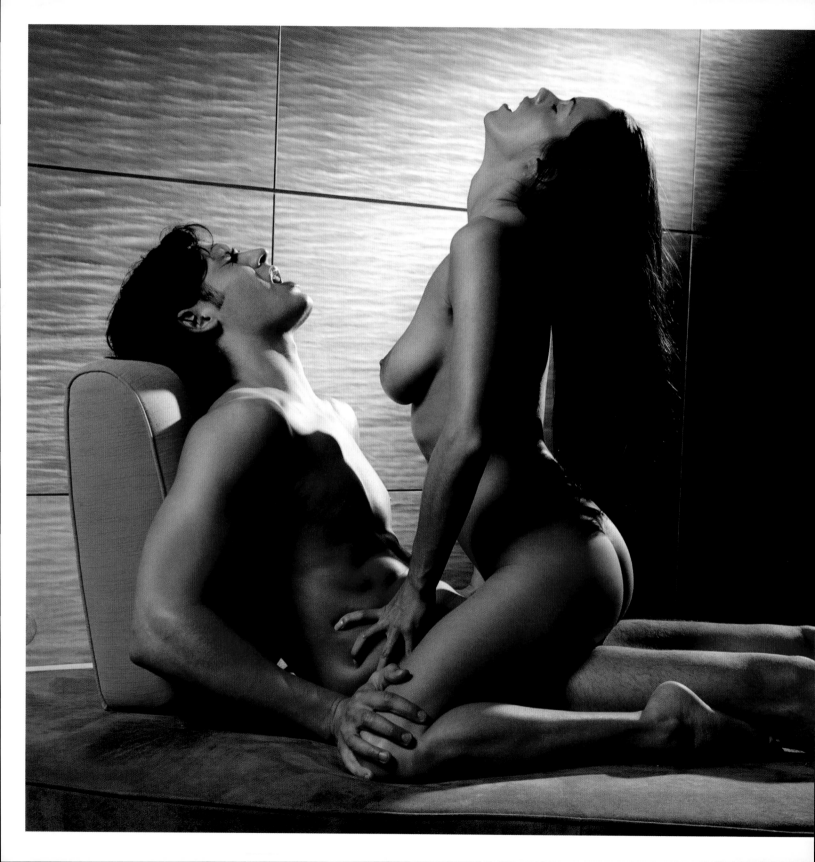

♂04 *Hot Positions for Intercourse*

Playing with new positions is one of the easiest ways to spice up your sex life and discover new orgasmic sensations. Sometimes you'll crave positions that offer shallow stimulation and clitoral contact, and other times you'll be craving deep penetration and acrobatic challenges. Whatever your desires, try the positions in this chapter and adjust them, as needed, to make them your own.

POSITIONS FOR SHALLOW OR CONTROLLED PENETRATION

Wait! Don't turn that page or skip to the next section. Shallow sex is perfect for:

Longer penises

Shorter vaginas

Longer lovemaking sessions

Full-intensity orgasms

G-spot orgasms

Clitoral orgasms

Coronal ridge stimulation

And a whole lot more...

Just as we erroneously assume that bigger is always better, we often mistakenly regard deeper penetration as a universal ideal. The reality, however, is that shallow penetration can be more desirable for a number of reasons. Not only are the most sensitive nerve endings of the vagina located in the lower third of the canal (sometimes referred to as the orgasmic platform), but other orgasm hot spots like the G-spot and the frenulum of the penis light up with pleasure at a shallow depth. The following positions are designed for mind-blowing orgasms through controlled-depth thrusting.

T-BONE

As your bodies form the shape of a T, this unique angle creates a sensation like no other with minimal exertion on your part. Perfect for those lazy Wednesday nights when you need your sexual fix but don't have the energy to hang from the chandelier.

Set It Up

She lies on her back with her knees bent and her feet spread apart flat on the mattress.

He lies on his side at a right angle to her body (to form the top of the T) and slides his body under the bridge of her bent legs.

She presses her hips up slightly as he slides in from beneath her. As they rock and thrust in rhythm, their fingers can dance over her clit or they can hold hands and gaze into one another's eyes.

Change It Up

A slight hip tilt by either partner can create a wave of new sensations as the head of his cock alternates between thrusting against her G-spot and pressing against her lower wall to provide anal stimulation. This not only changes her experience of the T-Bone, but he also benefits from the differing textures of her upper and lower vagina against his highly sensitive head and corona.

SEX TIPS FROM THE PROS

Ladies: Cross your legs and squeeze! Not only will you awaken the core muscles involved in orgasm, but as you squeeze his cock between your warm, wet thighs, the snug fit will create extra friction against his shaft and your tender inner lips.

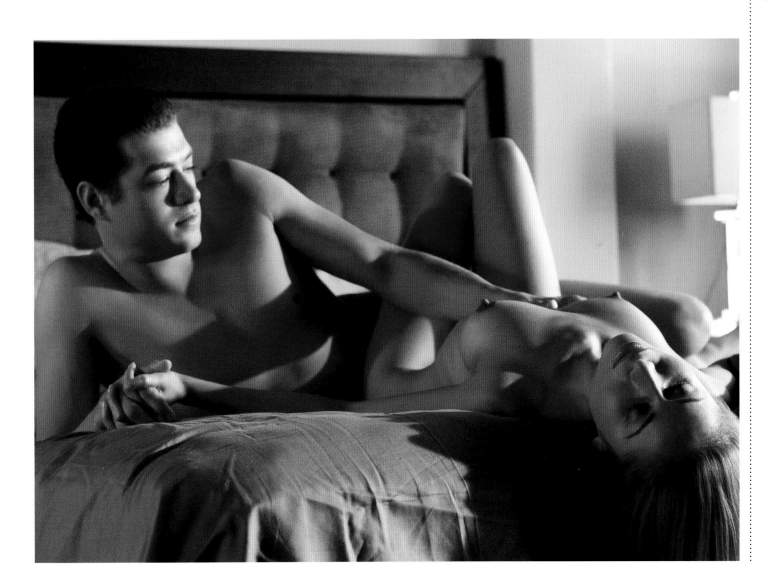

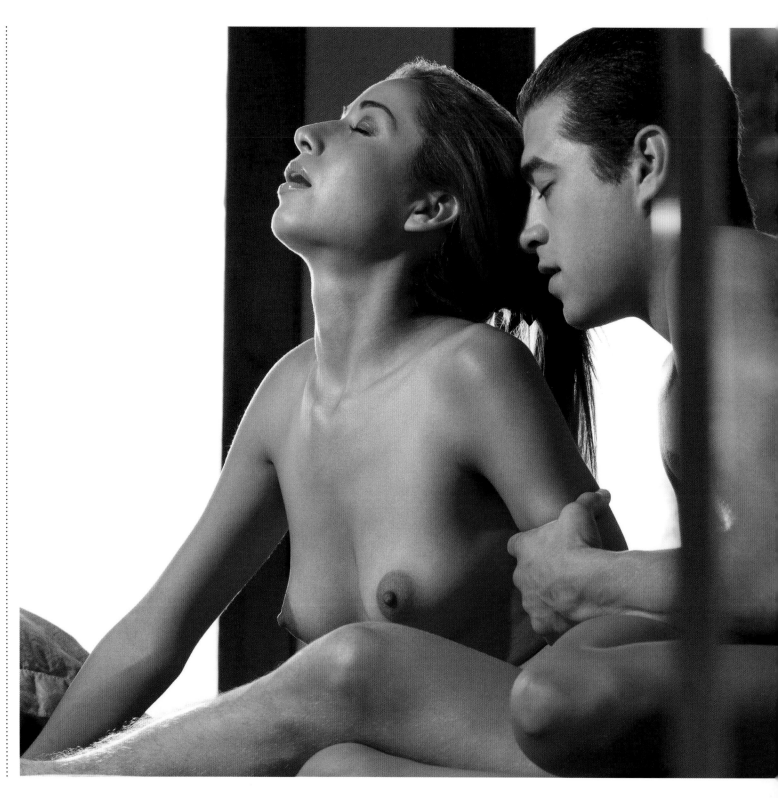

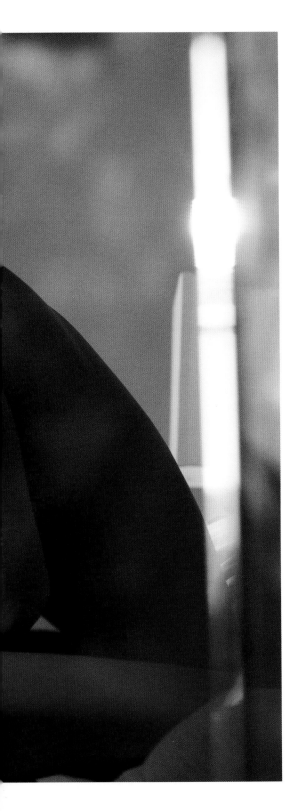

ROCK AWAY

A variation of the classic Scissors position, Rock Away is the ideal rear-entry setup for the often-elusive mutual orgasm during intercourse. He gets a tight grip around his shaft, and she benefits from a frenzy of friction against the entire length of her vulva.

Set It Up

He sits upright against the headboard with his legs outstretched.

She lies on her left side in his lap, facing away from him, with her butt pressed against his cock.

She scissors her legs open and slides her left leg under his right leg to straddle it between her thighs.

Leaning on her left elbow for support, she slides back onto his cock as his hands guide her hips.

She can pop over him back and forth, round her hips in an elliptical motion, twist sideways with care, or slide up and down to grind against his pelvic bone for extra friction.

Change It Up

You can transition to the challenging Side-Saddle Cowgirl position if he lies back and she sits upright into a squat or half-split position.

DR. JESS SAYS...

Rock Away leaves both of his hands and one of hers free to roam as they please. He can take control by grabbing her by the hips or reach around to fondle her breasts and stroke her clit. She can reach down to rub herself off or allow her fingers to wander around his legs, feet, balls, chest, and shoulders.

TITILLATION

This position is designed for uninhibited lovers and women who love to flaunt their best assets in his face. Though the depth of penetration may be shallower than other positions, he surely won't complain as she shoves her nipples between his eager lips and rounds her hips to envelop his throbbing head and shaft.

Set It Up

He lies on his back on the floor and pops his hips up as he slides his legs onto a bed or couch, leaving his ass a few inches in the air. Since much of his weight will be supported by his shoulders, he may want to place a few pillows beneath his neck and back for support.

She climbs atop on all fours, allowing her breasts to hang or press into his face.

She can control the angle, depth, motion and speed of penetration as well as the degree of contact between his face and her chest.

Change It Up

Ladies: Take complete control and tie his hands above his head as you tease him into an undeniable frenzy. Dangle your breasts just out of reach of his lips and pop your lips—the ones between your legs—just over the head of his swollen cock.

Gents: Spread her butt cheeks with your open palms and tease her ass by running a finger along her perineum between her fourchette and pucker.

UPRIGHT MISSIONARY

The ultimate shallow-penetration position, the Upright Missionary comes naturally and offers the benefits of intense eye contact, full upper-body views, and one of the tightest grips designed for bigger, better orgasms.

Set It Up

Apply lube to her vulva and inner thighs.

She lies on her back and he kneels over her with his legs on the outside of hers. He slides inside to get into position, then she closes her legs.

He holds the base of his penis as he barely slips in and out, and she squeezes her thighs together for extra friction.

Change It Up

Ladies: Wrap your thumb and index finger around the base of his shaft and move your hand in rhythm with his thrusts to form a human cock ring and intensify his orgasm.

BUTT BUDDIES

This challenging position has it all: The excitement of rear-entry, the mystery of "blind sex," the sensual bumping of butts, and the option for dual stimulation of her G-spot.

To facilitate entry, be sure to angle your hips upward so that his penis doesn't bend at an uncomfortable angle. Since penises can and do break (the tunic that encapsulates the spongy erectile tissue can tear), take care to alter the Butt Buddies position as needed.

Set It Up

She lies flat on her stomach with her head in the upper right corner of the bed.

He lies on his stomach on top of her with his head kitty-corner to hers in the lower left corner of the bed. His legs stretch out on either side of her, and their positioning deprives them of eye contact and exchange of facial expressions to facilitate "blind sex."

They both pop their hips upward far enough for his penis to angle backward comfortably and slide inside.

Gradually, they slide away from one another simultaneously and then back toward one another, allowing their butts to bump gently as they find their perfect rhythm.

Change It Up

Butt Buddies leaves the possibilities wide open for alterations and additions:

Ladies: Slide your hand down to your lower abs and press on your G-spot from the outside for dual stimulation.

Gents: Kink it up and press your feet into her cheeks or the side of her neck as you play with subjugating dirty talk.

Ladies and gents: Take advantage of the distance between you to lock into a hot, teasing role in which you're perfect strangers enjoying a casual but raunchy one-night stand.

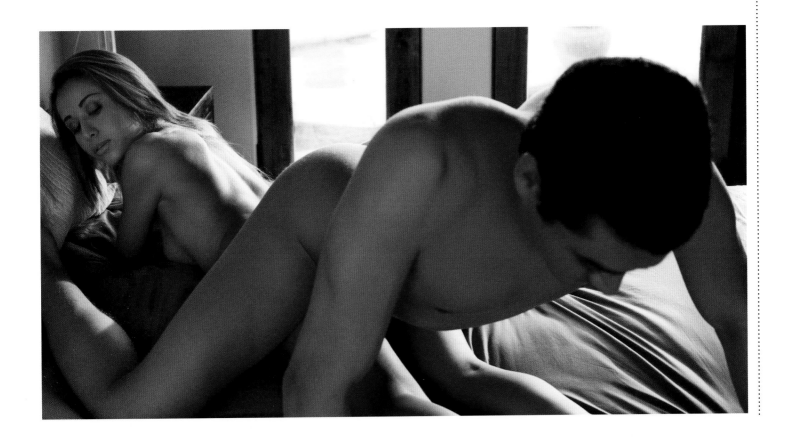

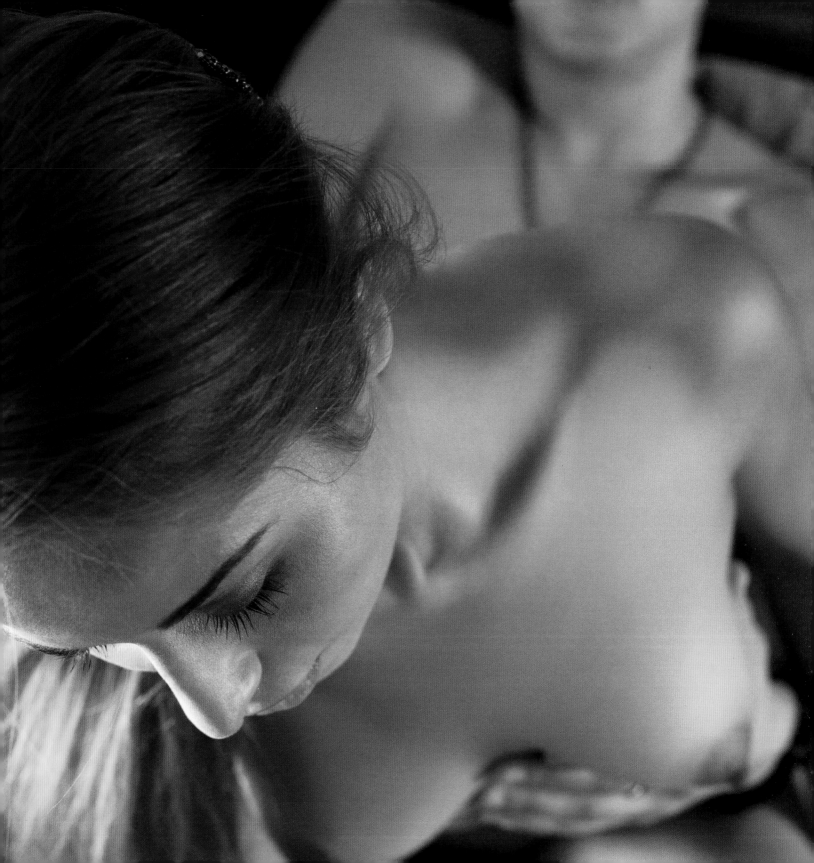

POSITIONS FOR DEEPER LOVE

Just like our appetite for food changes on a daily basis, so too does our desire for different types of sex. If you're in the mood for deeper penetration, play with these positions designed to access your hidden hot spots and breathe new life into your sexual repertoire.

BEND OVER BABY

This position is perfect for couples who want to experiment with a bit of power play. Her bent-waist stance ensures that her pelvis tilts backward for extradeep penetration. The rear-entry angle ensures activation of her sensitive A-spot as he squeezes the head of his cock into the tight space between her lower vaginal wall and her tender cervix.

Set It Up

He stands upright with his front side pressed against her backside.

She bends at the waist and pulls her hands behind her back as though preparing to be handcuffed.

He holds her by the hands and slides inside.

She can experiment with different hot spots by adjusting how far she bends down.

Change It Up

Perfect for a dominant-submissive role play, you can take this position to the next level with a pair of handcuffs, a little hair-pulling, and some light spanking.

Ladies: Spread your legs as you lean over and don't be afraid to bend your knees a little for comfort. Don't worry. He'll squat down to follow your lead.

PRIVATE DANCER

Take a page out of the professionals' book and arrange your bodies into a lap dance position for deeper, intense penetration. With your hands free, you're sure to find a few creative ways to bring yourselves to the heights of sexual ecstasy.

Set It Up

He sits on the edge of a couch, and she stands in front of him giving him a beautiful view of her backside.

With her feet (preferably in heels) on the floor in between his knees, she squats down over his entire length, allowing her body weight to rest in his lap for the ultimate in deep penetration.

Rolling her hips, she leans into him on the upstroke for full-body contact, but bends forward slightly on the downstroke to press his bulging head into her swollen G-spot. She can use her hands on his knees for support, and he can reach around to cup her breasts or guide her hips.

Change It Up

Ladies: Get even closer! Turn around and slide your knees on either side of his thighs on the couch as you press your breasts into his face.

DOUBLE DECKER

The Double-Decker is an all-time favorite for
women and men. Highly intimate, this position
facilitates manual stimulation to pleasure the
clitoris, breasts, prostate, and balls while
ensuring a tight fit around the base, shaft, and
head of his cock.

Set It Up

He lies on his back and she lies on top of him,
also on her back.

She guides him in, crosses her lower legs, and
tenses her pelvic floor muscles like she's sucking
an object into her vagina to squeeze his shaft
between her thighs.

She grinds up and down, pressing her fingers into
the top half of her vulva, and he pumps in tempo
with her movements while sensually rolling her
nipples between his thumbs and index fingers.

If it feels as though he is too close to slipping
out, he can slide a few pillows beneath his back
to assume a slightly more upright position and
increase his depth.

Change It Up

Gents: Place your hands under her hips and lift
her up slightly to pound more deeply.

Ladies: Hug your knees into your chest to relieve
stress on your lower back as you reach down
to fondle his balls and press into his prostate
through his perineum.

SIDESADDLE

Not only does this cowgirl-on-top position offer
full penetration, but the unique angle of her
body offers unparalleled contact with the sides
of her deep vaginal walls. If she likes to have her
cervix massaged, she'll fall in love—and he'll be
enraptured by the snug fit against the head of his
cock.

Set It Up

He lies down on his back along the edge of the
bed or on a couch.

She sits atop him with both feet on the floor,
varying her motions between up-and-down
strides, side-to-side Vs, and smooth semicircles.

SEXY SPLITS

Finally the flexibility she has developed in yoga class pays off! Perfect for supple bodies, the Sexy Splits position makes deeper penetration perfectly targeted as she winds her hips and curves her body. But he's not just along for the ride. He can plant his hands on her hips to guide his cock into her cul-de-sac or pull her close for some passionate kissing.

Set It Up

He lies on his back with his legs spread and she climbs on top, facing him.

Balancing on one knee between his legs, she places her other foot flat on the mattress next to his shoulder so that she assumes a partial lunge position. She can use her hands to help balance her body and he can offer additional support beneath her hips or butt.

Using her hands to guide his cock inside her, she rides away, curving her hips in large oval motions and grinding her vulva against his mons.

Change It Up

In keeping with the workout theme, she can slide her other foot up to land in a supported squat position with a simple swing of the leg. She can also change legs to ease the pressure on her hip and knee and alter the angle of penetration.

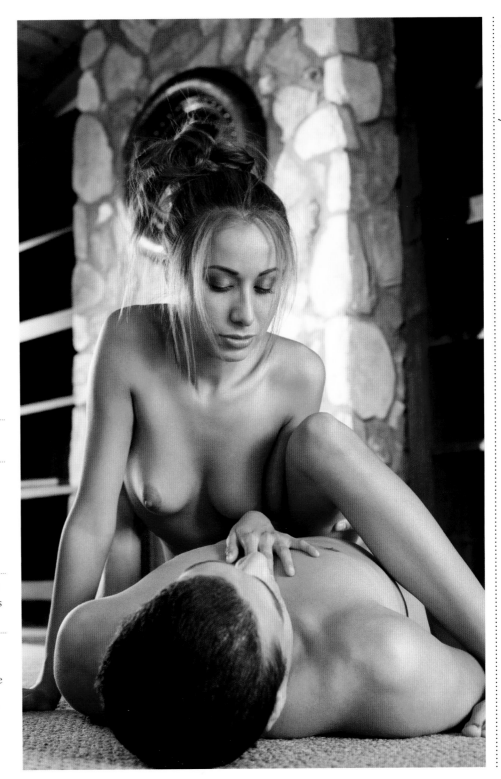

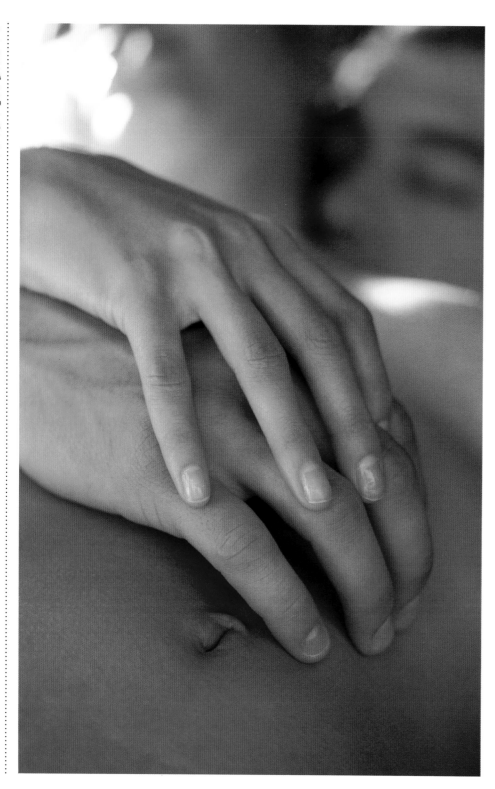

INTIMATE POSITIONS FOR DEEPER CONNECTIONS

If the eyes are the window to the soul, these intimate positions will inspire you to express your love to your soulmate in more ways than one. Making love (or just screwing) face to face offers a view like no other as her eyes roll into the back of her head, his gaze pierces you with desire, her smile signals the onset of the big-O, and his mouth falls agape with reflexive delight.

According to the cooperative eye hypothesis, the human eye is so essential to social and intimate interactions that it has evolved for the specific purpose of communication and cooperation. Some experts believe that this is why humans exhibit sharper color contrast in our eyes than other primates. However, if looking your lover in the eye during the throes of passion feels intimidating at first, you're not alone. Eye contact can induce feelings of passion even between complete strangers, and scientists attribute these feelings to the production of neurochemicals that stimulate adrenaline production. However, using this connection tool sparingly can actually work to your benefit, as studies suggest that you can sometimes be more persuasive in the absence of eye contact. Vary your gaze according to your personal comfort levels by looking your lover up and down with lust, closing your eyes to heighten your other senses, smiling coyly with fleeting gazes, or staring off slightly to express your overwhelming pleasure.

As you read through these intimate positions, tweak them as you see fit to make them your own.

FLAMINGO

This standing position lets you lock eyes—and hips—as you dance your way toward orgasmic bliss. You can alternate between shallow and deep thrusts to envelop his shaft and grind against one another's pelvic bones to rub her clitoral hood.

Set It Up

Stand facing one another as she lifts one leg to wrap her foot around his hip.

He bends his knees and slides inside.

Change It Up
Ladies: If you're feeling flexible, slide your leg all the way up his torso to open yourself up to him in the most personal of ways.

Gents: If you're feeling strong, pick her up and have her wrap her legs around your waist in the Stand to Attention position as you slide a little deeper.

ROCK 'N' ROLL

This position is designed for lovers looking to prolong their erotic session through minimal movement but maximum pleasure. The Rock 'N' Roll facilitates kissing, deep breathing, and naughty whispers in hushed tones.

Set It Up

He sits on the bed with his back against the headboard and his legs outstretched with a slight bend in the knees.

She sits on his lap facing him with her legs on either side of him and her feet planted on the mattress next to his hips.

He helps to pull her hips into him as she rocks against him, holding on to his shoulders. Alternatively, she can lean back between his legs, putting her weight on her hands on the bed.

Change It Up
Sit perfectly still in this position and take turns performing pelvic floor squeezes for a minute or two. The unique sensations of his hard cock pulsing against her swollen labia and the tight squeeze of her vagina wrapping around his shaft will prime you both for explosive orgasms.

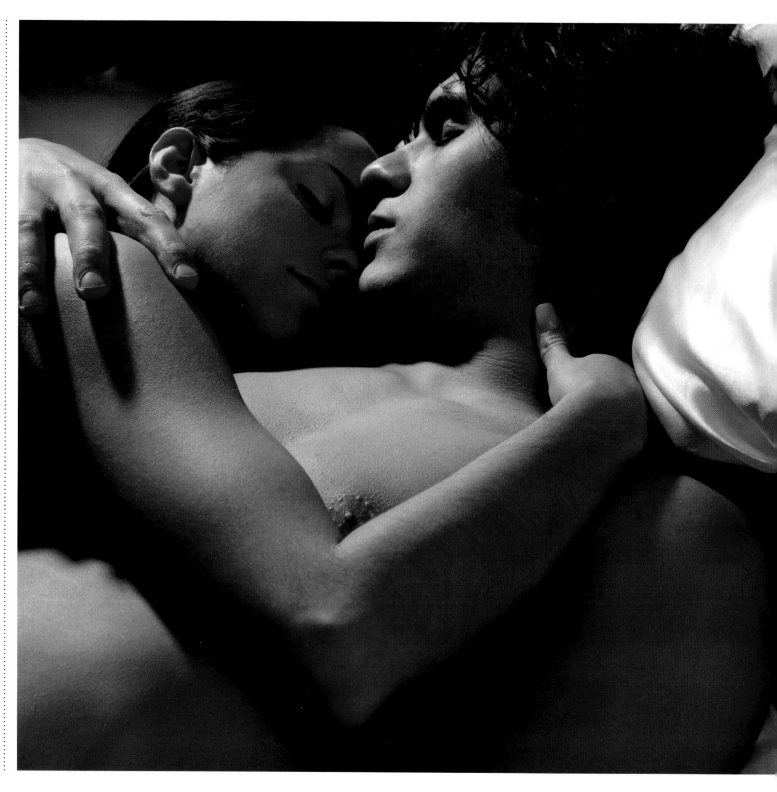

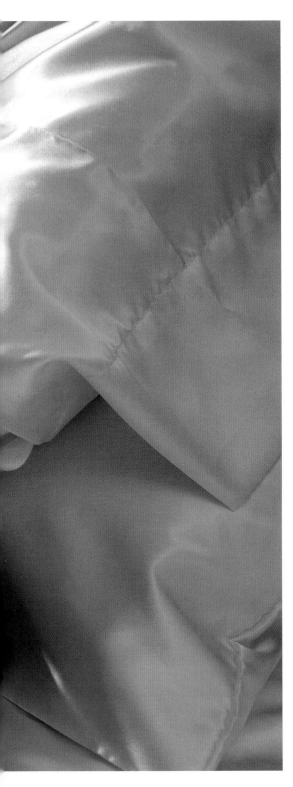

LOVERS IN ARMS

This position not only creates an intimate connection through full-body touch and eye contact, but it is ideal for transitioning from man-on-top to woman-on-top positions without missing a beat. A shallower reach allows for G-spot stimulation, and the side-by-side setup means your hands are free to wander and fondle as desired.

Set It Up

On a bed, lie on your sides facing one another.

To facilitate entry, she can slide her leg atop his body, wrapping it around his hips or waist.

Allow your hands to wander. Run them through your lover's hair, caress her face, trace your fingertips down his back, or simply wrap your arms around one another in a loving embrace.

Change It Up

Ladies: As you slide your leg up toward his chest and down toward his feet, the angle of penetration will alter the sensations for both of you. You can also squeeze your legs together for more clitoral stimulation or slide your fingers between your bodies for direct contact.

Gents: To increase the depth of penetration and skin-on-skin grinding, slide your upper leg between her legs, allowing her to grind against your pelvic bone.

MARRY ME

Romance is still alive, but orgasms make it better than ever! In this position, he not only gets down on one knee, but the angle of penetration ensures that the tightest part of her vagina wraps around his sensitive corona as his hard shaft massages her sensitive clitoris.

Set It Up

He gets down on one knee and slides the other leg out to the side in a bent position. The foot of the bent leg should be planted firmly on the mattress.

She also kneels on one leg and throws her other leg over his bent knee. If there's a significant height difference, she can use pillows beneath the knee she's kneeling on.

He slides inside and they thrust toward one another in opposing rhythm.

Change It Up

Try this one from behind in a modified doggie-style: He remains in the same position, but she turns and places her hands flat in front of her. Keeping one knee planted, she throws her other leg back over his to create a welcome invitation for his eager cock.

POSITIONS FOR CLITORAL STIMULATION

Almost any position can be modified to include manual stimulation of the clitoris, and many couples find that mutual orgasms become more common when they use their hands or a toy during intercourse. There are, however, a few hands-free positions designed to directly stroke the clitoris during penetration to produce powerful orgasms as your lips wrap tightly around his happy cock.

THE CAT

The CAT (Coital Alignment Technique) position offers a simple twist on the classic missionary pose. It provides clitoral and vaginal stimulation, ensures a tight grip around the shaft, excites the prostatic nerves, and requires no acrobatic skill!

Set It Up

She lies on her back and the man lies on top, with his legs on the outside of hers. When they're both ready, he slides inside, pressing his body against hers.

He then shifts his body upwards along hers (he can rest his hands/arms beside her head) so that the base of his penis and pelvic bone press firmly against her clitoral hood and pelvic bone.

She wraps her feet around his calves if desired.

Play with synchronized rocking and rubbing movements as opposed to in-and-out thrusting.

DR. JESS SAYS . . .

Some women find intensified pleasure in squeezing their legs together during the CAT to create greater friction and tension. This squeezing sensation can also heighten sensation in the penis as her lips tighten their grip around his shaft.

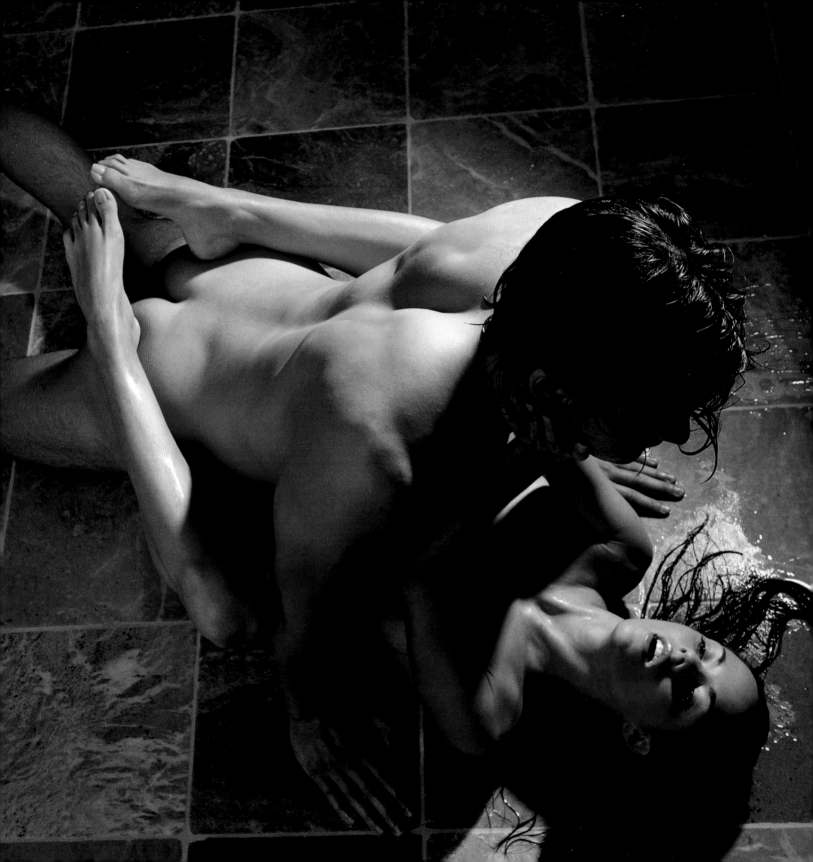

SCISSORING

This is the ideal position for women who love full-clitoral contact. She uses his thigh as a grinding pole to rub her entire clitoral complex while he pumps away to his delight.

Set It Up

You both lie on your sides facing one another but with heads at opposite ends of the bed.

She scissors his upper leg between hers as she rolls slightly onto her back.

He pumps inside of her as she grinds her vulva against his thigh for clitoral stimulation.

SWINGER

This sexy pose not only allows you to admire one another's bodies face to face but also provides the clitoral friction most women need to experience orgasm during intercourse. But it's not all about her! He gets a prime view of her bouncing breasts while plowing deep inside of her and watching her gasp with pleasure.

Set It Up

She lies on her back with her legs hanging off the side of the bed or couch and her feet touching the floor.

He kneels or squats between her open legs (atop a pillow, if necessary, to adjust for height) and slides inside.

She wraps her legs around his body as he leans forward slightly.

As he pumps, she pulls him in closer with her legs and grinds her clitoris against his mons. To intensify the pleasure, he rolls his hips upward as he pumps in and out to rub her clit with the firm surface of his pelvic bone.

SEX TIPS FROM THE PROS

If you love clitoral play during intercourse, just do what comes naturally to you. Scissoring may be perfectly designed for clitoral grinding, but if you experiment with a range of positions, you'll find lots of opportunities to rub yourself off against his pelvic bone, leg, fingers, and even the hard base of his shaft.

EASY ON THE BACK, KNEES, AND OTHER INJURED PARTS

Not all sex positions require acrobatic skills, and earth-shattering orgasms can be had in the most gentle of positions. Whether your sex life has been affected by temporary aches and pains or more serious, permanent injuries, small adjustments can help you to make sex more comfortable. From the simple addition of a pillow beneath your knees to a new angle that reduces the pressure on your hips, practical adaptations are sometimes necessary to maximize pleasure.

As you adjust your bodies and positioning to suit your body's unique needs, remember that comfort is elemental to sexual enjoyment. There is no one-size-fits-all position for neck/shoulder/back injuries, so listen to your body and respond accordingly. These pleasure-packed positions offer modifications for those with joint issues, limited mobility, and various injuries. They're great even if you don't have an injury!

THE CURVE

This rear-entry, side-angled position is designed for women with back injuries and men who have knee, hip, or wrist injuries that keep them from positions in which they have to support themselves on top.

Set It Up

She lies along the side of the bed, presenting her voluptuous ass to him over the edge of the bed.

He stands on the floor next to her or kneels (if kneeling is not problematic) on a few pillows to ensure an appropriate height for penetration.

He presses the tip of his cock against her labia, but she curves her back and slides over him to ensure comfort.

He reaches around to press his fingers against her clitoris as she squeezes her legs around the base of his shaft.

Change It Up

She can wrap her feet right around his butt to pull him into her and take greater control of the thrusting motion.

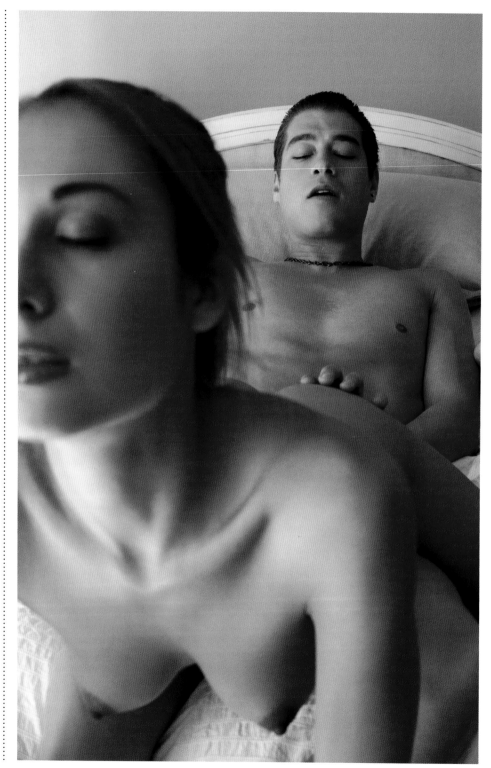

REVERSE EAGLE

Designed for men with back or knee injuries, the Reverse Eagle is not just an injury-modification position. It may become your new favorite with its capacity for frottage (sensual rubbing), deep pumping, and the added bonus of anal play.

Set It Up

He lies on his back with pillows beneath his knees, back, and neck as needed.

She straddles him, facing his feet and sending her legs back widespread with her feet on either side of his shoulders.

She places her hands between his legs for support and rolls her butt in a semicircular motion as her outer lips grip his cock from base to tip.

They simultaneously stroke one another's perineums, breathing deeply into toe-clenching climaxes.

Change It Up

If the weight of her body causes strain on his hips or lower back, she can relieve some of this pressure and create some hot visuals between her legs by squatting over his cock instead.

DOWNWARD DOG

This erotic version of Downward Dog lets her rest flat on her stomach as he protects his back by adjusting according to his own comfort level. Not only is this one of the top positions for female orgasms, but the adaptable positioning works well for a variety of injuries.

Set It Up

She rests on all fours and he kneels behind her to enter her in the classic doggie-style position.

Slowly, she lowers herself onto the bed with a few cushions beneath her hips, and he follows with his cock buried deep inside.

She lies still as he angles his body in the most comfortable position possible for hard, deep thrusting. His legs can be in between hers, or one or both can be outside of hers. Depending on whether his back pain arises in flexion or extension, he can adjust his positioning accordingly.

She slides her hand beneath her mons and allows the weight of their bodies in conjunction with his thrusting to stroke her clitoris into a throbbing climax.

HAPPY SPOONS

The classic spoon position is perfect for knee, back, or neck injuries and can be enhanced with a few well-placed pillows beneath your neck or knees. The intimacy of front-to-back full-body contact coupled with easy access to her clitoris makes this a go-to position for the most experienced of lovers.

Set It Up

Both partners lie on their sides with his chest against her back.

Use a rolled-up towel or pillow beneath his neck for comfort and allow her to determine the curve of her body if she has a back injury.

He enters her from behind.

She guides his hand down to her mons and clitoris for additional manual stimulation of her most sensitive pleasure organ.

Change It Up

Create a bent-spoon pose by curling your legs upward into a cozy fetal-like position. Not only does this change the feelings associated with the angle of penetration, but it also allows him to thrust using his thighs as opposed to his hips.

FOR THE ACROBATS AMONG US

Sometimes we're in the mood for lazy, Sunday-morning sex, but other times the challenge of a new sexual experience can boost our adrenaline and create new sexual highs. Experiment with the following poses and make alterations as you see fit to maximize your safety and your hedonistic experience.

Sex positions are not bucket-list items, and you don't have to check off a minimum number to be a great lover or enjoy a hot sex life. However, since our interpretations of pleasure and pain can change with time, do revisit new positions every so often, even if you didn't love them the first time around.

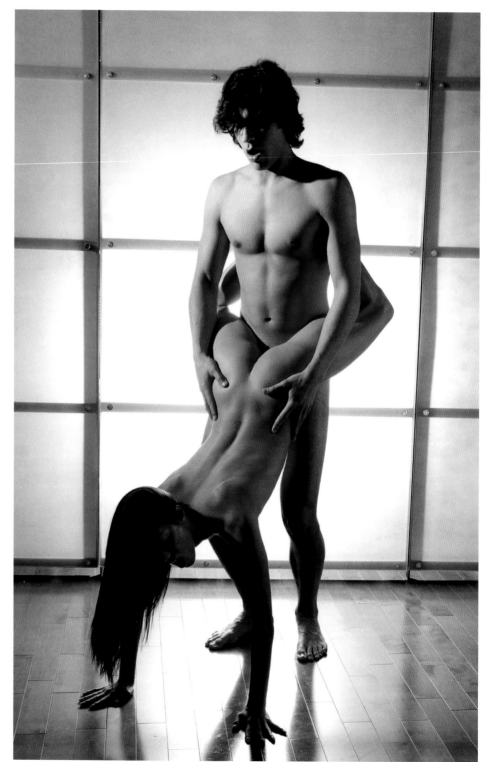

MILE-HIGH CLUB

Tighter airline restrictions may reduce the chance of ever joining the traditional Mile-High Club, but you can take your sex life to new heights with this pose that's like flying. He gets a hot view of her lips around his cock as he piles into her A-spot with fervid delight.

Set It Up

She kneels on the floor with her forearms resting on the bed in front of her.

He stands behind her between her legs, lifts her hips into the air, and slides in as her legs fly out on either side of his hips.

She flexes her abs to ensure that her back doesn't arch into an uncomfortable swan-dive position.

Change It Up

Try this position on the couch, but let her upper body rest on a padded arm to ease the pressure on her lower back.

RISK TAKER

The thrill of the Risk Taker position lies in the physical pose as well as the danger associated with the challenging positioning. As he slides inside from an inverted squat position, her fourchette rubs against his sensitive spongy tissue and frenulum, and she is forced to lie perfectly still to protect his most prized asset.

Set It Up

She lies on her back with her legs spread slightly and bent up into the air. Propping her hips up with a few pillows may help to facilitate entry.

He squats over her, facing away and resting his butt on the backs of her lower thighs.

He bends forward and she angles her pelvis upward so that he can slide inside and pump up and down.

She fondles her own sweet spots while he reaches down and plays with his balls or her pucker.

Change It Up

Up the ante and try the Risk Taker with him doing a partial handstand on the floor next to the bed. He can place his feet on either side of her shoulders on the bed. Her butt should rest just on the edge of the bed, and she can clasp her hands around her ankles to hold her feet in the air.

PULL-UP

This position requires a bit of forethought with the mounting of a door-frame chin-up bar, but the possibilities for creative sex poses are almost limitless, so the minor installation will be well worth it. Not only is this challenging position good for muscle tone, but as she wraps her legs all the way around his body, the Pull-Up creates the perfect pose for the deepest thrusting possible.

Set It Up

Install a chin-up bar in a load-bearing door frame. Easy as pie, right?!

She grabs the bar overhead with both hands and loosely wraps or rests her legs on his hips. He slides inside of her, allowing her legs to now wrap around his waist.

He partially supports her weight as he plows inside, and she allows her body to swing slightly, creating a whole new momentum.

Change It Up

Ready for a real challenge? Test his fitness by switching roles and letting him hang from the bar as he thrusts inside of her from behind. Placing a stool beneath his feet provides temporary rest and relief to facilitate this modified position.

TOPSY-TURVY

Another yoga move comes in handy in the
bedroom! A supported shoulder stand creates
an inverted position designed for a snug grasp
coupled with added sensation over his super-
reactive head.

Set It Up

Lying on her back, she uses her hands to support
her lower back as she lifts her legs and butt up
into the air with her toes pointing toward the
ceiling.

He kneels in front of her and helps her feet up
onto his shoulders to alleviate the pressure on
her neck. For mutual support, he holds on to her
thighs, and she holds on to his.

He slides inside, angling his shaft downward
ever so slightly.

Change It Up

Try this one in a full handstand position. He
might need a stool to adjust for height.

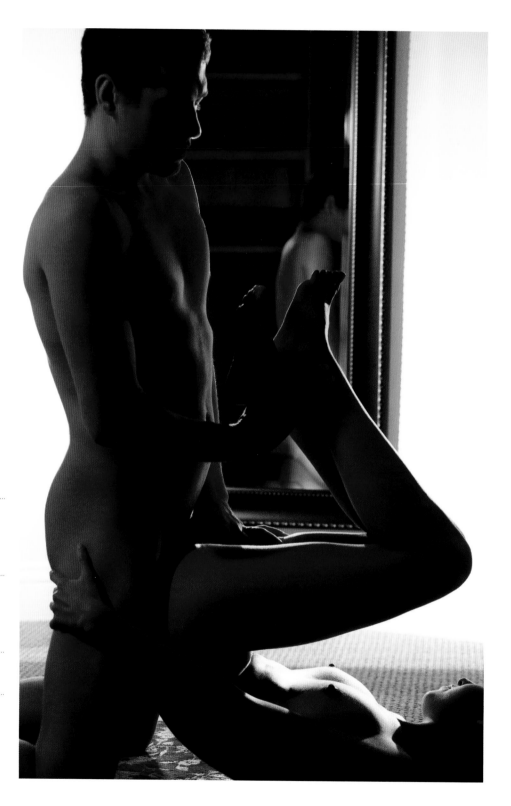

TECHNIQUES AND ENHANCEMENTS

Hot sex isn't just about finding the right position. After all, if it's the motion in the ocean that keeps you coming, you'll want to learn a variety of techniques to keep the fires burning. And while the only way to be sure your lover is satisfied is to ask for suggestions and feedback, bringing a few new techniques into the bedroom is sure to inspire some memorable experiences and meaningful conversations.

Sometimes we're in the mood for lazy, Sunday morning sex, but other times the challenge of a new sexual experience can boost our adrenaline and create new sexual highs. If you're looking to contort your body into pretzel-like versions of wild animals, you may want to get warmed up with a bit of stretching or yoga earlier in the day.

However, you'll likely find that as you become more turned on, your body will naturally fold into more challenging positions with greater ease thanks to the chemical changes associated with arousal that increase palliative functioning. Accordingly, if you're looking to try something new and challenging, get yourself all riled up beforehand to ensure a safe and pleasurable experience.

Sex positions are not bucket-list items and you don't have to check off a minimum number to be a great lover or enjoy a hot sex life. However, since our interpretations of pleasure and pain can change with time, do revisit new positions every so often even if you didn't love them the first time around. You may find that a position that left you wanting more a few months back is now a sure-fire path to orgasm.

The upcoming positions are designed to help you discover new orgasmic spots and angles, but they also offer an added bonus: as you flex, bend, tuck, and lunge, you'll also be burning extra calories, increasing flexibility, and strengthening your muscles. And because exercise and sexual functioning are positively correlated, you'll be killing two birds with one stone!

Experiment with the following poses and make alterations as you see fit to maximize your safety and your hedonistic experience.

TIPS FOR WOMEN ON TOP

Some women enjoy the sensations of riding their lovers but are intimidated by the thought of being physically exposed from the waist up or feel uncomfortable being in the driver's seat. Blindfolding him (or yourself) and lowering the lights can help you to overcome any physical self-consciousness, and developing a positive body image will not only make you more attractive but also increase your sexual satisfaction. If being on top is a new or rare venture, begin in small doses when you're highly aroused and you'll find that your inhibitions will dissipate in no time!

Mount him tonight, as he lies on his back, and try one of these moves:

The Classic: Bounce up and down on his cock from base to tip.

The Cat Curl: Place your palms next to his shoulders and arch your back like a cat to curl your hips backward, then pop your hips back and forth in a semicircle.

Booty Circle: Sit up straight and roll your hips to trace a large circle. Glide the bottom half of the circle along his body and the upper half in the air as you allow his shaft to slide out slightly.

Rocking Horse: Sit all the way down and rock your hips from front to back. Picture yourself sensually riding a rocking horse for this move … It's weird, but it works!

Sexy Squat: Squat over him and let him watch your inner lips suck him slowly from the lowest point of his base to the very tip of his cock. Alternate between 5 slow strokes and 10 quick ones to bring him to the peak of arousal.

On Your Knees: In a kneeling position, lean backward and pump up and down.

Table Top: Get on all fours and whisper dirty thoughts in his ear as you lower your hips over his cock.

Quick Change: Alternate between ten very shallow pumps and ten deep ones, pressing your lips and lower thighs into his hips/pelvis. Experiment with other rhythmic patterns as well.

Hip Roll: Roll your hips in semicircles popping your butt toward his toes and then up toward his head.

Sidewinder: Curve your hips in a circular motion from side to side while you slide up and down his shaft.

Booty Pop: Turn around to face his feet and pop your butt backward and upward.

Slide: Close your legs and lie flat against him as you slide up and down his cock. Rather than popping up and down as you might if you were straddling him, slide your entire body up toward his head and then back down toward his feet. The movement is minimal, but it packs a pleasurable punch!

Upward Dog: Once he's inside you, slide your legs between his and squeeze your thighs together as you ride him, supporting yourself with straight arms on either side of his chest.

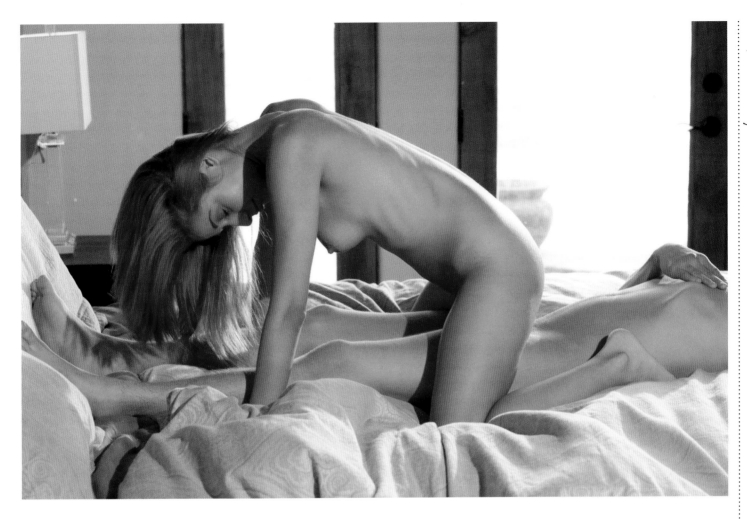

Ringer: Lean back slightly and wrap your thumb and index finger around the base of his cock for a tighter grip as you ride him.

Good Vibes: Turn around to face his feet and surprise him by rolling your favorite toy along his balls while you pop up and down his shaft.

Selfie: Forget about his needs entirely. Ride, rub, grind, and rock yourself off as he enjoys your natural moans, reflexes, and facial expressions.

Triangle: Thrust your hips forward (toward his head) as you lower yourself over him. Glide back against his abs ever so slightly (toward his feet) when you reach the deepest point before stroking back upward. This triangular move not only provides extra friction against his frenulum and your clitoris but also massages the full width of the deepest point of your vagina.

Hot Profile: Give him a sexy view as you shift your body to the side. Just be careful not to bend his penis as you slide both legs on one side of his hips.

Self-Love: Cup your breasts in your hands or fondle your nipples to put on a sexy show.

Sexy Squeeze: When you need a little break or simply want to change things up, slide yourself all the way to the base of his cock and clench and release your pelvic floor muscles around him several times.

Wet That Whistle: Spread the love by reaching down between your legs and spreading your wetness around while you ride him. If he likes a little ball play, sweep your fingers all around them using your natural juices, and be sure to remind him just how good it feels for you.

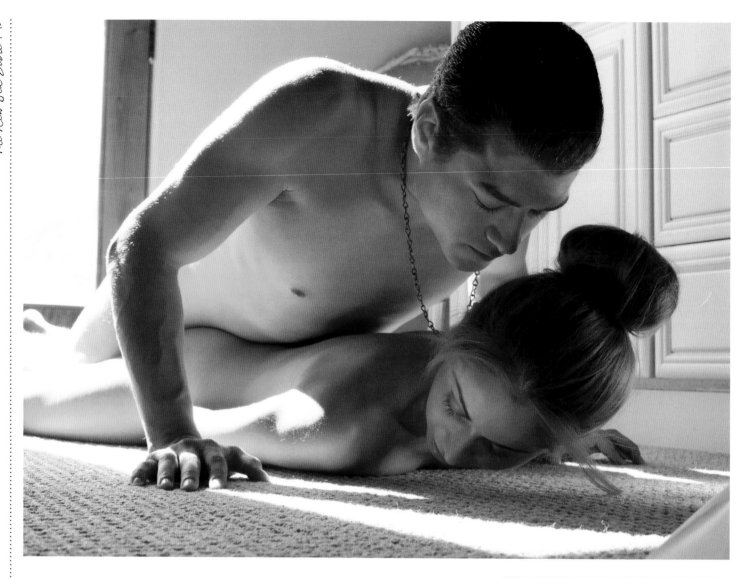

TIPS FOR MEN ON TOP

Being on top may seem like a natural position for most men, but the repetition of your basic pumping and thrusting can lead to boredom in the bedroom. Moreover, most women don't reach orgasm from the classic in-and-out motion alone, and if you've come this far, you obviously prioritize her pleasure. Play with and alternate between some of the following movements to keep things sizzling and take your sexual prowess to the next level.

Lady Vee: When she is lying on her back, lift her legs into the air to increase the depth of penetration.

Tempo: Slide inside of her as slowly as possible, allowing the sensitive nerve endings of her inner lips to be awakened by the texture and curve of your cock. Once you're completely buried inside of her, hold still and perform a few pelvic floor squeezes/Kegels (see page 24) to mimic the orgasmic contractions of orgasm.

The Hover: Hover your body over hers as you slide in and out. Whisper in her ear, "You make me so hard. Your body drives me wild. I can't get enough of this. Do you like that?"

Classic Roll: Roll your hips in an exaggerated circular motion as you thrust. Try this movement in any position to alter the angle at which your shaft rubs her vaginal walls.

The Circle: Slide your cock halfway inside of her and roll in a wide circular motion without thrusting. Try it at a shallow, medium, and full depth to find and stay focused on her hot spots.

Shoulder Press: Grab her by the ankles and press her feet against your shoulders as you plow into her deeply.

Thigh Screw: Lube up your cock and slide it between her thighs to get her all riled up. She'll be begging you to put it where she wants it most.

It's All in the Hips: Flip her on all fours and immobilize your pelvic area as you pull her onto your cock with your hands on her hips. If she likes it rougher, grab her by the butt cheeks.

Pull and Play: During the early part of your sex session, pull out and tap the upper half of your cock against her vulva, using your hand to control placement and pressure. Slide the head of your cock up and down along her labia to awaken the nerves of the clitoral legs and bulbs and then press or tap the underside of your cock (and frenulum) against her clitoral head and hood.

Shallow Groove: Thrust into her using only the head of your cock for a minute and then alternate these shallow pumps with some slow, deep ones.

Leg Lift: Bend one of your legs to the side as you thrust to discover greater depths and new angles.

Curls: Tilt your hips up slightly when you're on top and decrease your depth of penetration to curl your head against her G-spot.

Grind: Gently grind your pelvic bone against the very top of her vulva to stroke her clitoral shaft as you slide in and out.

Lean: Sit her up against the headboard and lean back as you pound into her to pump against her A-spot.

Surprise: Keep her favorite vibrating toy handy (make sure it's charged!) and press it into her mons or clit to take her over the edge.

Shallow Jackhammer: Pump in and out as quickly as possible using only the upper third of your cock.

Wave: Undulate your entire body on top of her in a wave-like motion.

Breast Caress: This one takes a bit of coordination but is well worth the practice, as her brain will react with excitement to unexpected and disparate sensations. Thrust firmly into her at a fast pace while you very gently caress and encircle her breasts with the backs of your fingernails.

PULSE, SQUEEZE, AND MORE!

Combine your sexy positions, sensual movements, and oral techniques with these additional enhancements and you'll be all set for a lifetime of happy endings. Developed to amplify your body's natural reactions to sexual stimuli, mix and match these add-ons with a variety of new moves and old favorites to create an infinite number of sexual experiences and longer, stronger, more satisfying orgasms.

Pulse!

Pulsing sensations are a mainstay of bigger, better sexual finishes, as they mimic the powerful contractions that both men and women experience with orgasm. As you pulse against your lover's sweet spots, the brain and body naturally recall the pulse-like spasms of orgasm, which can be felt in the vagina, uterus, prostate, anus, penis, and pelvic floor. Some people, however, report feeling similar pulse-like impressions across their entire body: from their hips and thighs to their tongues and nipples. Orgasmic waves can spread like wildfire, so don't limit your focus to the obvious zones as you pulse away before and during orgasm.

You can add the pulse to any move, technique, or position, and allowing your own drive and desire to inspire you will make it all the more exciting! Here are a few suggestions to get you started:

Pulse your lips (either set!) around the base of his shaft or corona as he nears orgasm.

Slide your thumb over her clitoral glans or hood and pulse gently.

Press two fingers into his perineum and pulse every half second.

Pinch her nipples between your thumb and index finger and pulse firmly.

Pulse your middle finger against the outside of his pucker.

Press your palm into her vulva and pulse away, increasing your speed and pressure as her arousal builds.

Squeeze!

When it comes to erogenous zones and all of our juicy sexual parts—particularly those that are composed of erectile tissue—a well-timed squeeze can work wonders. Though we tend to associate squeezing or pinching with pain, science as well as widespread personal accounts reveal that moderate pain can actually be pleasurable. This is because the same reward circuits of the brain light up during both pleasure and pain, and our interpretations of these sensations sometimes overlap. As you experiment with perfectly placed squeezes during sex play, proceed gradually, beginning with very gentle squeezes of larger areas, or have your lover show you just how she likes it. You may want to try the following squeeze techniques during foreplay, oral sex, or intercourse:

Squeeze the base of the penis with your thumb and finger in the shape of an "okay" sign to harden his erection.

Squeeze her nipples between the sides of your fingers.

Connect your thumbs behind his scrotum and bring your index fingers around the base of his penis against his lower abs. Squeeze snugly to form a human cock-ring.

Squeeze her inner labia between your lips.

Squeeze your thighs together to activate the muscles connected to your pelvic floor.

DR. JESS SAYS . . .

The way you breathe has a significant impact on your sexual and orgasmic response. And though each of our bodies is unique, many people report that deep, slow breathing intensifies their orgasms and can even result in multiple climaxes.

Tingle

Full-body orgasms are often described in terms of the tingling sensation we experience in the most surprising of places, and we can encourage that tingly feeling to spread the love across the entire body. Make your lover's body tremble with a featherlight touch using the tips of your fingers, the backs of your fingernails, or the warmth of your gentle breath against any body part you can access. If you're lying on your back beneath him during intercourse, run your fingertips softly down his spine and lick your lips as you exhale slowly over his earlobes. If you're thrusting inside of her from behind, trace the backs of your nails against the small of her back or the nape of her neck. Replace fondling and kneading with a tingle-soft touch during oral sex or a makeout session and watch your lover's body quiver with delight.

Twist and Twirl

A simple twist can be added to almost any sexual activity to awaken new nerve endings and keep your lover guessing. Twist your tongue over the head of his cock during a blow job, or twirl your hips to the side slightly while lying on your back to press your cervix into his corona as he slides inside. Play with new sensations without changing positions as you twist your legs to the right or left during intercourse or twirl your tongue in opposite directions during cunnilingus to build her anticipation for the unexpected.

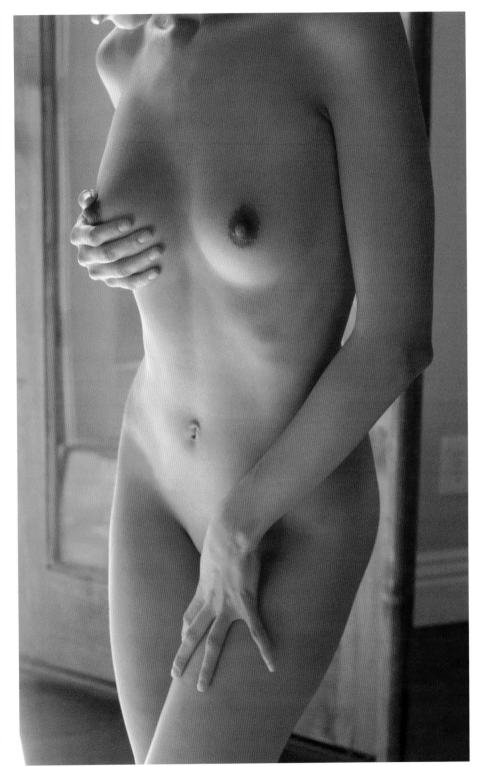

DR. JESS SAYS . . .

Though sex during pregnancy might just be the hottest sex of your life, you do want to take precautions to protect your changing body. Certain positions (like the CAT, page 110) can cause discomfort and others (like a shoulder stand) may not be doable, so be sure to make adjustments to suit your body. If you find that cervical pressure is painful or uncomfortable, you may want to reduce the depth of penetration, and though sex during normal pregnancies is perfectly healthy, check with your medical practitioner if you have any concerns.

SEX DURING PREGNANCY

Though sex is almost always central to getting pregnant, our culture's erotophobia (a general fear of and negative response to sex) often desexualizes pregnant women and mothers in an irrational manner. This is a shame, as pregnancy and motherhood are not only intensely sexy, but sex during pregnancy can be an extraordinary experience. Changes in hormone levels during pregnancy can actually boost your libido, and though orgasm may be slightly more elusive during the first trimester, many women report experiencing more intense climaxes during the second. Some women say their bodies and their genitals in particular are more responsive during pregnancy, and many men say their attraction to their partners skyrockets during this stage.

That being said, every woman's experience with sex during pregnancy is unique and you can expect your feelings and desires to fluctuate over the ten-month period. While some women report feeling hornier than ever, others find that the body changes, weight gain, and general exhaustion wreak havoc on their libido.

Erica and Richelle are best friends who gave birth weeks apart but tell two very different stories. Erica craved sex throughout the entire course of her pregnancy and loved the pleasure derived from her new swollen breasts. Richelle, on the other hand, describes pregnancy as "the antidote to sexiness" and was grateful that her husband was on the same page. The bottom line is that there is no universal experience of sexuality during pregnancy and you shouldn't feel pressure to conform to any standard of abstinence or indulgence.

As your body changes, you may have to make modifications to your sexual routine, including technical and positional shifts, and this exploration can result in a broadening of your sexual horizons. Some fun positions for pregnant women include the following.

FRISKY BUSINESS

She stands facing the wall with her legs spread and her hands against the wall above her head. He stands behind her and slides inside. As her baby bump grows during pregnancy, this position may need to be adjusted to create space between her stomach and the wall. She has several options, including adding a slight bend in the waist, kneeling on a chair, or using an open doorway instead of the wall.

QUEEN BEE

She lies on her left side supported by pillows beneath her knees, ankles, or shoulders. He kneels behind her and helps her to bend her right (top) knee upward as he enters from below. This is the perfect positions for adding a "reach-around," which he can tailor to her specific preferences: a stroke of the clit, a gentle tug of the Venus mound, or the addition of some intense vibrations are sure to make this bee buzz with pleasure!

LEGS UP

She lies on her back on a high pile of pillows with extra support beneath her hips. He kneels between her thighs and lifts her legs up to cradle them against his forearms as he penetrates from below. As she lifts her legs into the air, she may find that the pressure on her cervix is too much to handle. If this is the case, she can press the soles of her feet into his chest to control the depth of penetration.

FAQ: MY WIFE IS SEVEN MONTHS PREGNANT AND
WE BOTH HAVE HEALTHY SEXUAL APPETITES. I'M
A BIT CONCERNED, HOWEVER, ABOUT WHETHER I
MIGHT HURT MY BABY DURING SEX. CAN I POKE HIM?
SHOULD I BE MORE GENTLE? AND IS SEX REALLY SAFE
WHEN SHE'S THIS FAR ALONG?

Sex in pregnancy is always an issue that many couples want advice on from their doctors.

Partners can have sex throughout the entire nine months as long as there are no complications with the pregnancy such as:
1. cervical issues
2. preterm labor
3. possible miscarriage
4. bleeding in pregnancy

OB/GYNs usually state that as long as the pregnancy is proceeding normally you can have sex as often as you like. The cervix is a barrier between the vagina and the uterus where the fetus is growing. This helps to prevent infection and harm to the fetus. The baby is also protected by the amniotic sac in the uterus which contains fluid. Also the uterus protects the baby, as it is a strong muscle. Most sexual positions are considered safe practice in pregnancy, however, as the pregnancy progresses it may be become more uncomfortable to maneuver during sexual intercourse. Other positions to consider include lying sideways next to your partner or positioning yourself on top or in front of your partner.

Jessica Shepherd, M.D., M.B.A.
Assistant Professor OB/GYN University of
Illinois at Chicago
Founder of Her Viewpoint

REAL PEOPLE, REAL SEX

"Pregnancy can actually inspire new sex acts. My pregnant wife was riding me and looked down at her belly and said, 'That must be awkward for you. I can fix it!' Then she turned around into Reverse Cowgirl." —Shane, 42

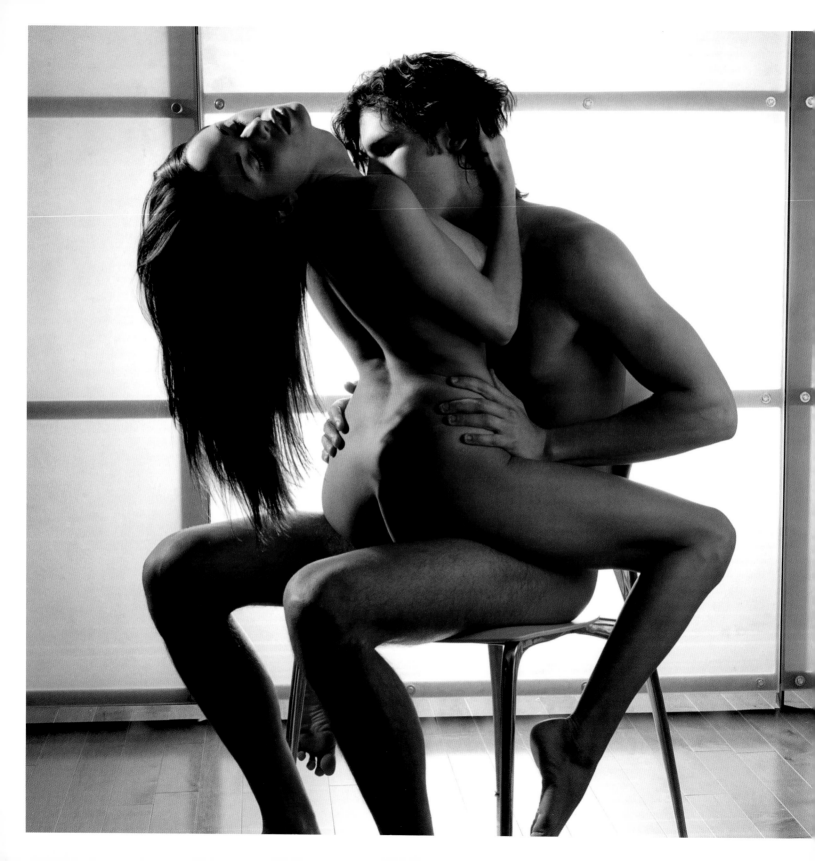

05 *The Big Ohhh!*

Orgasms, in all their glory, are a central feature of sex. For many, orgasms are the ultimate sexual indulgence, as they leave us feeling relaxed, fulfilled, and overwhelmed with gratification. But part of what makes orgasms so glorious is the fact that no two are the same. Dr. Ruth Westheimer suggests that orgasm is simply a reflex, like a sneeze, but this seems rather understated, as a sneeze doesn't overtake your body so intensely that your center of reasoning and behavior shuts down in response to a rush of pleasure.

THE FEMALE ORGASM

Over the past ten years, I've collected descriptions and definitions from workshop participants, and their responses illustrate the range of experiences with orgasm:

"It's just like a sigh, but a bit better."

"It feels like a total body experience that culminates with a massive burst of hot lava from the penis."

"At that moment, nothing else matters."

"Like fluttering wings over my eyelids so the whole world is perfect and hazy."

"The most sumptuous of desserts."

"Two thunderbolts and a trickle."

In the coming pages, I cover various types of orgasms, but it is important to note that none of these categories is perfectly defined or mutually exclusive. In fact, orgasms do not fit neatly into categories based on a particular technique or body part. Though we may *experience* different types of orgasms, we cannot accurately categorize them into a universal system. For example, thanks to the imperfect seminal work of Sigmund Freud, we often view clitoral orgasms as oppositional to vaginal ones when in fact they can be one and the same.

Accordingly, what follows is a generalization of orgasm types based on both anecdotal descriptions as well as scientific research with regard to brain and nerve activity. It is of paramount importance to preface this information with a reminder that there is no pleasure hierarchy. Your experiences of orgasm are of the highest order, regardless of how you get there or how your body reacts. You may want to experiment with different approaches to orgasm, but there is no value in checking "types" of orgasm off a sexual bucket list, as the associated pressure can detract from the pleasure of sex as an experience.

From a subtle sense of relief to an earth-shattering wave of full-body pleasure, the female orgasm is a true shapeshifter in that no two experiences are the same. Similarly, the path to orgasm varies widely, and despite what you may read in your latest women's magazine, there is no surefire method to produce mind-blowing orgasms. Techniques offer guidance and inspiration, but ultimately, it is variety, experimentation, and familiarization with one's own body that eventually lead to the climactic sensations of toe-curling pleasure.

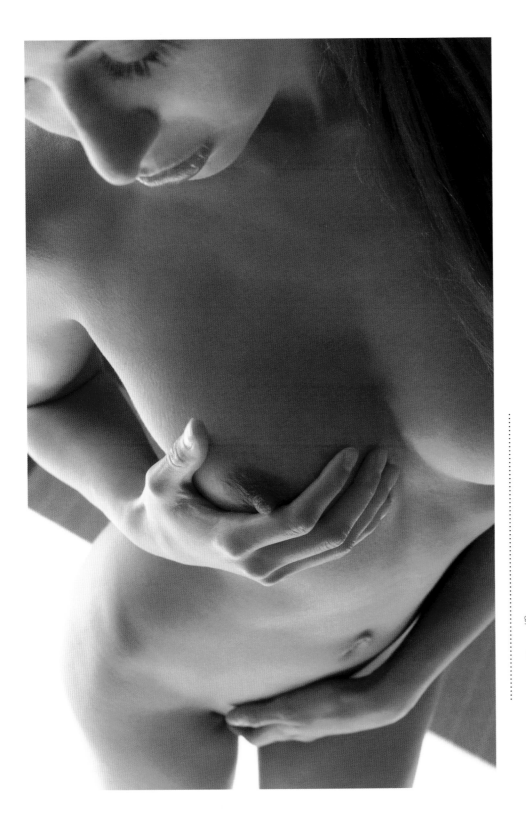

FAQ: HOW DO I KNOW IF I'VE HAD AN ORGASM?

Ellen Barnard, MSSW, of A Woman's Touch Sexuality Resource Center in Madison, Wisconsin, explains that if you feel a sense of release and pleasure, you've probably had an orgasm. "An orgasm is a buildup of muscle tension in your genitals (and often legs) that peaks and releases with a rush of pleasurable feelings that are sometimes centered in your genitals, and maybe other parts of your body. You may feel pulsations of the pelvic floor muscles that surround your vagina and anus at the same time as that feeling of hitting peak tension and release."

CLITORAL ORGASMS

Clitoral orgasms are considered the most common of all orgasms for women, and most ladies report that they require some stimulation of this sensitive organ in order to climax. Some women experience clitoral orgasms during intercourse, but many positions don't provide enough friction or stroking to take her over the edge. There is good news, however, as there are a few simple solutions.

As you'll recall from Chapter 1, the clitoral complex is composed of many parts both inside and outside of the body. You can stroke its legs and bulbs through the labia, rub its shaft via the hood, stimulate its erectile tissue through the shallow walls of the vagina, or apply direct pressure to its highly innervated head. Many of us have a tendency to get hyper-focused on the head of the clitoris, and this is one reason why the female orgasm can be so elusive. Pressing, flicking, and encircling the clitoral head can be arousing, but it can also be annoying and even uncomfortable at times. Most women report that its sensitivity and pleasure capacity fluctuates depending on how aroused they are, and some opt to forgo direct touch in favor of indirect stimulation (e.g., pulling on the skin of the mons to stroke the hood over the erect shaft) at the peak of arousal.

As always, the best way to figure out what works is to play with yourself and share your findings with your lover. Our bodies are constantly changing, so what spikes your arousal one day might have the opposite effect a few weeks later. Our continuous sexual evolution highlights the need for ongoing experimentation and serves the purpose of keeping sex fresh and exciting.

Because the clitoral complex is so large and shares many connections with the entire pelvic region, women experience clitoral orgasms from a wide array of stimulation techniques. If you're looking for new approaches or have yet to experience a clitoral orgasm, try these techniques on for size:

Run a finger (or your partner's tongue) over the clitoral hood to stroke the erect shaft. Increase your pressure and pace until you reach a rhythm of two to three strokes per second.

Rub your vulva over any firm surface, allowing your body weight to create extra friction. The arm of a padded couch or a rounded staircase banister should do the trick.

Slide a flat or wide vibrator like the We-Vibe Touch or the Hitachi Magic Wand back and forth over the entire vulva in the motion of a swinging grandfather clock pendulum.

Use the palm of your hand or a toy to apply firm pressure to the entire vulva as you squeeze your legs together and flex the muscles of your pelvic floor.

Slide your favorite toy inside and circle it around the shallow opening of your vagina to stimulate the erectile tissue of the clitoris. Double your pleasure by tugging firmly on the lower part of your mons to stroke your pulsating shaft.

Pinch your outer lips around the head of your clitoris with your index and middle finger as you slide them in a rhythmic motion from top to bottom. Alternate between stroking up and down and rolling your fingers over your entire vulva in a large oval with lots of pressure.

During intercourse, grind your lower mons against any firm surface you can find: a mattress, the edge of your bed, your fingertips, his pelvic bone, his thigh, a toy, etc.

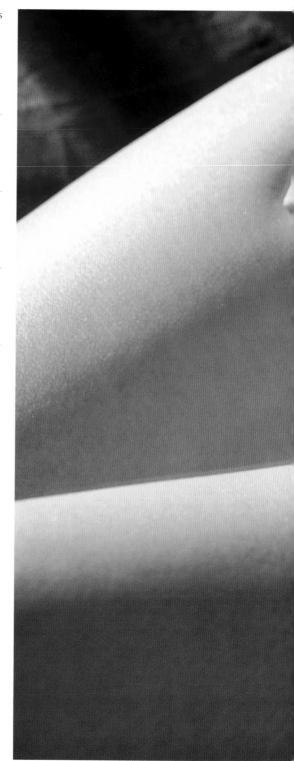

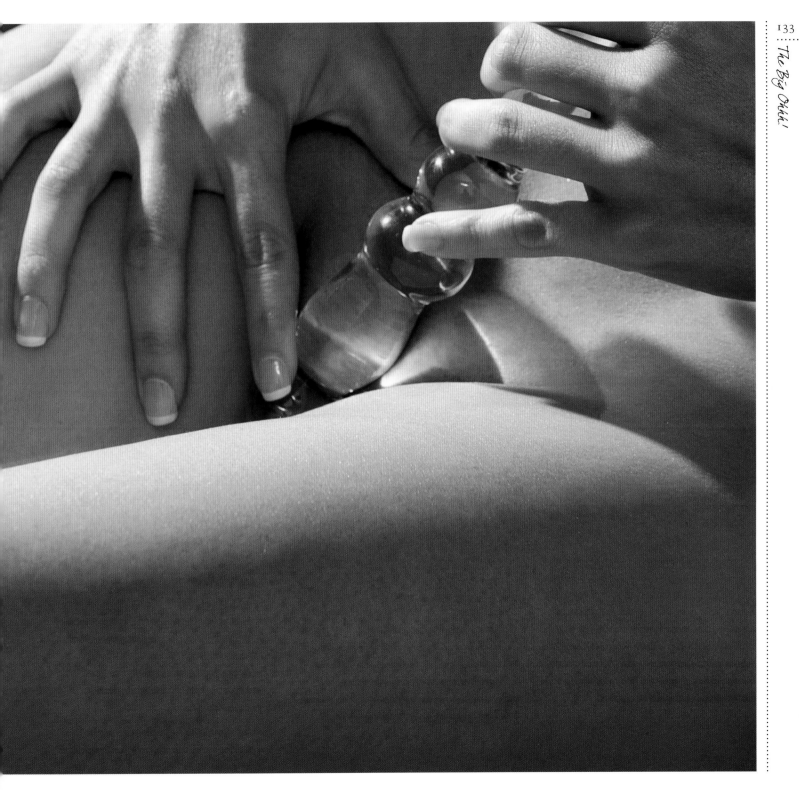

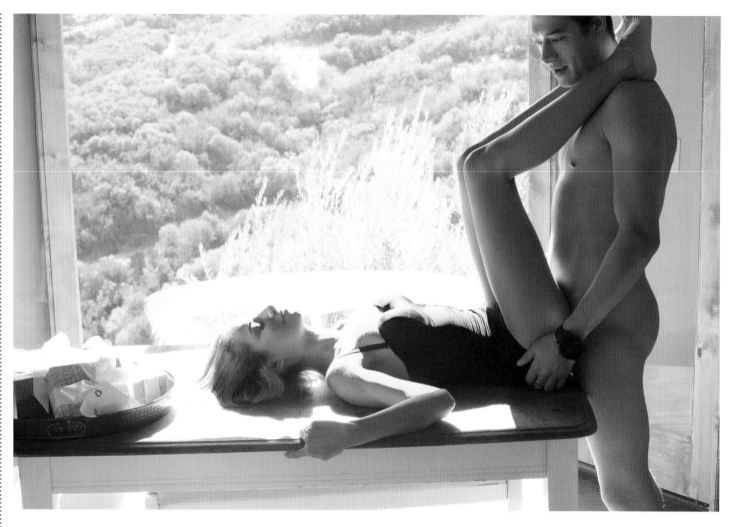

VAGINAL ORGASMS

Vaginal orgasms are not invariably distinct from clitoral ones, and there is a great deal of overlap between these interconnected erogenous zones. Research suggests that vaginal penetration alone results in orgasm for approximately one-third of women, but this figure may be misleading, as the vagina and clitoris are not only close neighbors but are, in fact, connected by a number of nerve pathways and muscular structures.

For this reason, some experts believe that all genital orgasms are clitoral in nature on account of the corollary stimulation through the vagina. Others disagree and point to laboratory observations of brain activity during orgasm, which suggests that different areas are activated depending on which part of the genitals are being stimulated. But even these researchers acknowledge that there is some overlap, suggesting that perhaps it doesn't matter how we *label* our orgasms—only that we *enjoy* them.

If you take pleasure in having your vagina caressed, massaged, penetrated, or touched, try these techniques to take your orgasms to new heights:

Swirl the object of your choice (a tongue, penis, toy, or finger) around the opening of your vagina in a circular motion against its walls. Gradually increase the depth as you spiral to the back (toward your cervix), pressing into the sides as they swell with pleasure.

Use a toy to apply firm, pulsing pressure to her A-spot at the very back of her vagina toward her stomach wall.

Combine vaginal penetration with some backdoor fun by sliding your index and middle finger inside the vagina and pressing down toward the back wall. Gently pinch these fingers together with your thumb against her perineum.

Alternate between shallow, slow, gentle thrusts and deep, hard pumping, as the outer part of the canal tends to be sensitive to light touch whereas the deeper zone is often more reactive to pressure.

Squeeze and release your pelvic floor muscles every half to full second during penetration to increase blood flow and orgasmic response.

Her cul-de-sac can be highly reactive to temperature, so try alternating between warm and cool by dipping a toy in water of varying degrees.

G-SPOT ORGASMS

G-spot orgasms also overlap with clitoral and vaginal orgasms, as the area known as the G-spot is accessible through the front wall of the vagina and is located in very close proximity to the legs of the clitoris. Both scientific and anecdotal accounts of G-spot orgasms, however, suggest that they are distinct from other experiences of pleasure. Women often report that a G-spot orgasm feels different from a clitoral one, as they experience sensations of bearing down with their pelvic floor muscles as opposed to the tenting effect from clitoral stimulation.

Pioneer sex researchers Beverly Whipple, Ph.D., and Barry Komisaruk, Ph.D., have also discovered that vaginal, cervical, and G-spot stimulation activates different parts of the brain via four different nerve pathways that innervate the clitoris, vagina, and cervix. What is most exceptional about this differentiation is the fact that the vagus nerve bypasses the spinal cord, allowing even those diagnosed with complete spinal cord injury to experience pleasure and orgasm via the cervix.

If you want to explore the orgasmic capacity associated with your G-spot, you may want to experiment with the following techniques:

Curl two fingers into the vagina and press them into the upper (stomach-side) wall in a "come hither" motion.

Slide three fingers into the vagina and sweep them back and forth like windshield wipers against the upper wall.

Use a toy designed for G-spot stimulation or try the Magic Banana, which has a flexible loop that curves perfectly into this spot and also doubles as a Kegel exerciser.

Slide a penis inside from the front, but insert it only halfway. Round her hips back to press his corona against her G-spot.

FOR SEX GEEKS

For many years, medical professionals believed that a spinal cord injury indicated the end of one's sex response and experience of orgasm. However, Dr. Whipple and Dr. Komisaruk found that pleasurable and orgasmic sensations can migrate to various parts of the body including the ears, lips, breasts, and nipples. Over half of women can reach orgasm after a spinal cord injury, and less than a quarter say they are less satisfied with their sex lives.

Shelli was diagnosed with complete spinal cord injury after a serious car crash at the age of eighteen, but her sex life is still red-hot. "Because of a lack of vaginal sensation, my husband and I have had to be more creative to enhance my sexual experiences, but it also makes it more fun. I have found that I have other very sensitive erogenous zones and in fact had one amazing orgasm from stimulation on my breasts alone!"

Men with spinal cord injury can also experience erections, ejaculation, and orgasm post-injury. Through the stimulation of a range of body parts, some people describe genital-like sensations even if they do not experience feeling in this area. What the research with spinal cord injuries and sex teaches us is that orgasmic sensations need not be relegated to the genital region. Our bodies are massive conduits of pleasure and their full exploration can result in heightened response and pleasure.

SQUIRT! FEMALE EJACULATION

There seems to be a great deal of misinformation floating around about female ejaculation, but the expulsion of fluid from the urethra is a fairly well-documented phenomenon. Not only do early sexual texts, including *The Kama Sutra*, reference women's expulsion of fluid during sex, but the latest research reveals that the skene's glands, which are a part of the G-spot and drain into the urethra, are homologous to the prostate gland in men. Female ejaculation, like male ejaculation, is a sexually induced reaction that may or may not coincide with orgasm.

Mainstream porn may tout this "spraying" sensation as some sort of sideshow trick, but in reality, the fluid expelled is usually less than a teaspoon in volume and generally doesn't squirt across the room. Its contents are similar to male prostatic fluid, and while some describe it as sweet tasting, others say that the taste is rather subdued.

The skene's glands are embedded in the spongy tissue that surrounds the urethra between the vagina and the bladder. It is therefore common for women to feel as though they have to pee when the G-spot is stimulated through the vagina or the abdominal wall. Many of us tense up, contract our pelvic floor muscles, or cease stimulation altogether in reaction to this sensation, warding off orgasm entirely.

While it is possible to expel small traces of pee, emptying your bladder before sex play can help to alleviate this concern. In the event that you do release a small amount of urine due to pressure on your bladder and urethral sponge, rest assured that this fluid is also harmless and, like ejaculation, often goes unnoticed during sex.

Female ejaculation is not a sign of femininity or sexual responsiveness. Similarly, a wetter reaction does not necessarily indicate a more enjoyable experience or greater skills as a lover. Our culture is patently competitive, but sex shouldn't be a competition.

If you want to experiment with ejaculation, try it on your own first to help reduce the pressure of performance and embrace your own reaction without focusing on any particular goal:

Get yourself all riled up in a manner that is familiar and effective.

Sit back against the headboard with your legs bent and your feet flat on the mattress.

Curl a finger into your vagina and pull up toward the wall of your stomach. Press into the upper wall as you feel the tissue begin to swell.

As you become more aroused, continue to curl your finger on the inside while you press down on your bladder through the outside of your stomach. This dual stimulation provides a light squeezing sensation against the G-spot by internal and external means.

If you feel like your muscles are inclined to bear down as though you're forcing air out of your vagina, exaggerate the feeling and release your pelvic floor muscles.

Breathe deeply and increase the pressure against your G-spot from both sides.

Embrace your body's reactions and don't focus on ejaculating. If it happens, that's great! And if not, simply embrace the experience of exploring your body and discovering new pleasure zones.

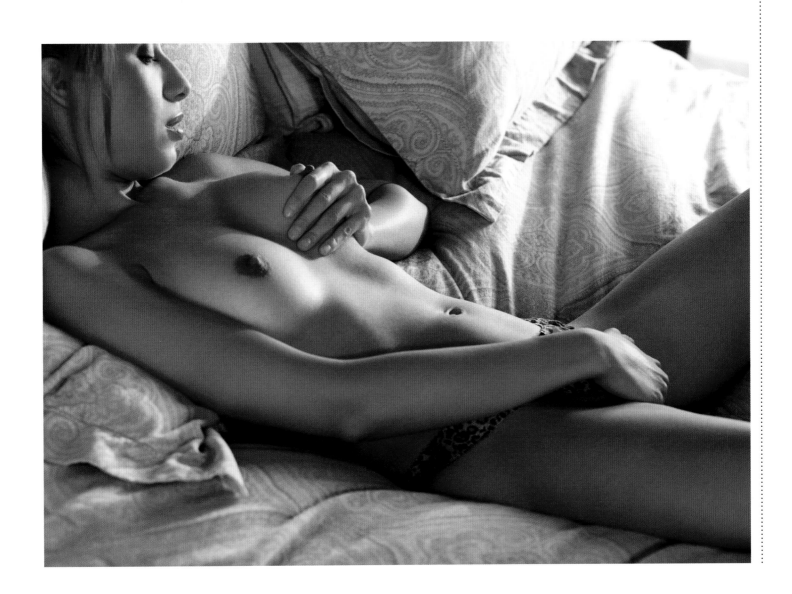

SEX TIPS FROM
THE PROS

Doing your Kegel exercises on a regular basis
will help you to take control of your sexual
and orgasmic response. Alternate between
performing a few sets of medium-paced
squeezes and releases for one minute at
a time and "elevator" Kegels in which you
gradually contract and release as slowly as
possible. (See page 24 for more on Kegels.)

FANTASY ORGASMS

Sex is often pigeonholed into a physical act
involving the genitals, but the reality is that the
hottest sex happens between our ears. Our most
thrilling and erotic memories do not often pertain
to wild sex acts, positions, or techniques but to
the intensity of our mind's involvement in an
experience. As we develop greater comfort with
our own sexuality and genuinely embrace our
desires, we find that hot sex is less about aesthetics
and more about an experience of intimacy,
connection, and uninhibited exploration.

So powerful is the mind's hold over our
sexuality that some people can actually "think"
themselves off through fantasy and breath work.
Technological advancements provide evidence
that some women can have hands-free orgasms.
Sex researcher Barry Komisaruk and his team
at Rutgers University have observed this type of
orgasm in the lab and studied the brain's reactions
using MRI technology.

Though only a small percentage of people report
reaching orgasm through fantasy alone, you
may want to experiment with the power of your
mind to increase arousal and expand your sexual
horizons. Allowing your mind to wander into
unchartered territory can help you to recognize
and benefit from your most genuine fantasies and
untapped desires.

We often stymie our sexual thoughts because
we believe that certain fantasies are off-limits
for social, political, religious, and even ethical
reasons; however, sexual fantasies that contradict
our real-life personalities, ideologies, and
experiences are perfectly normal. For example,
though no woman wants to be raped, this is a
common sexual fantasy for many of us, as we take
pleasure in the submission, victimization, and
targeted aggressive desire. Fantasies are not an
indication of mental health or real desires, as they
allow us to teeter on the edge from a safe place:
our minds.

In order to embrace your fantasies and allow them to carry your arousal to new heights, you first have to allow them to run wild and accept that they are healthy and normal. There is a clear distinction between thinking about a sex act and compulsively seeking out a sex act that causes harm to ourselves or others. Rest assured that no matter how outlandish your fantasies may be, they likely fall in the range of normal. Not only are fantasies associated with healthy sexual functioning, but a lack thereof is connected with low levels of sexual satisfaction and even sexual dysfunction. As long as you can differentiate between fantasy and reality, embracing your desires and allowing your body to respond to their natural progression may be just what you need to experience high levels of arousal from thought alone.

Barry R. Komisaruk (Ph.D., Distinguished Professor of Psychology), whose groundbreaking research reveals some of the most important insights into the process of orgasm, reminds us that there is no universal formula for fantasy orgasms:

> "We are still acquiring data on this phenomenon and to our best knowledge at present, the similarities in brain response during fantasy versus clitoral self-stimulation are greater than the differences.
>
> The women whom we studied told us that they just discovered serendipitously their ability to have orgasms by thought. They described a variety of strategies, not necessarily erotic (e.g., a loved one whispering in their ear, walking along the beach on a warm sunny day, moving energy through their body). So it seems to be the same basic method as that in which we learn to move our fingers—difficult to teach to others; we have to teach ourselves."

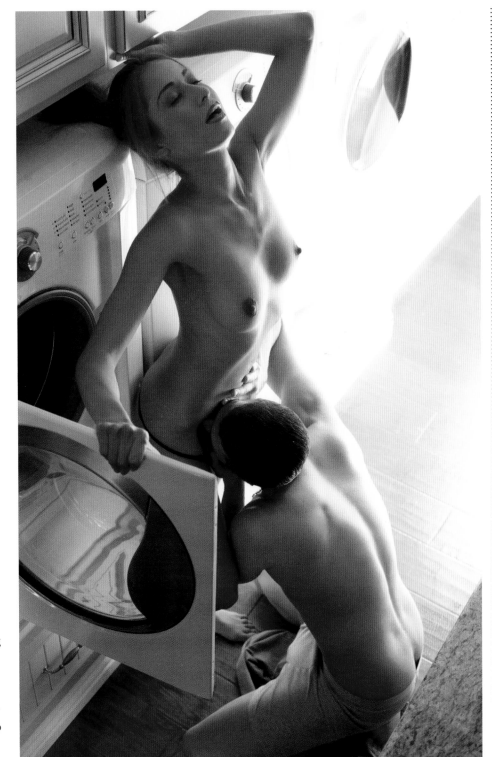

REAL PEOPLE, REAL SEX

"Hey guys! Could you stop treating my breasts like dough that requires kneading? Ouch! But seriously, less is more—especially when we're just making out." –Katy, 25

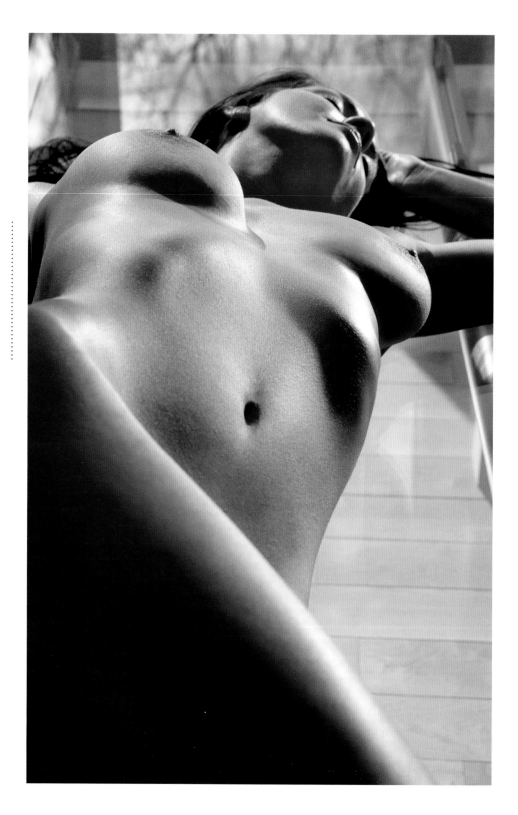

BREAST ORGASMS

Breasts are often at the forefront of sex play—and for good reason! Not only are they soft, round, and beautiful to look at, but they are a primary source of pleasure for many women and men. In fact, some women can actually reach orgasm from breast and nipple stimulation alone! This may be attributable to the fact that the genital sensory cortex in the brain, which is the same region impacted by stimulation of the vagina and clitoris, is activated through nipple play. Scientists hypothesize that these shared neurons release oxytocin, which induces pleasure and relaxation and spikes to peak levels just before orgasm.

But the nipples are not the only sensitive part of the breast. Many women pinpoint the area right above the areola as the most responsive to sexual touch. And the breasts change considerably during arousal, increasing (temporarily) in size and sensitivity. Ask her to show you how she likes to be touched at various points in her arousal cycle, or put these tried-and-true techniques to the test:

Start on the outer edges of the breasts using the backs of your fingers and circle your way slowly into the center. Roll her nipples as lightly as possible between your thumb and index finger.

Prime her for a night of passion using nothing but your breath. Tease her nipples gently until she's begging for you to suck them into your warm, supple mouth.

If she is sitting upright, curl your tongue under the soft fold on the underside of her breasts as you trickle your fingers along the sides.

Tell her how much you love them! Genuine compliments are food for the sexual soul: "Your tits are perfect. I can't get enough of them. I want to spray my hot come all over them!"

Nibble on her nipples as she approaches orgasm. Her pain thresholds can double at this point in the arousal cycle, and the overlap between pleasure and pain responses in the brain can heighten her orgasmic awareness.

Slide your lips over her nipple and twirl your tongue gently around her areola while you cup her breasts from below.

Pinch and release her nipples every half second right before she comes.

Squeeze her breasts gently together as you run your face, nose, and tongue between them.

Encircle her nipples with ice cubes or popsicles as you lick up the tasty mess.

FAQ: THIS MAY SOUND WEIRD, BUT MY WIFE IS STILL BREASTFEEDING AND I'M NOT SURE WHAT TO DO WITH HER BREASTS DURING SEX. SHE USED TO LOVE HAVING THEM FONDLED, BUT NOW I FEEL AWKWARD.

Since every woman's body responds differently to pregnancy and breastfeeding, the best way to find out what she wants is to ask her. Some women prefer not to have their nipples sucked while they're still nursing due to lactation and hypersensitivity, while others enjoy the heightened sensation. There is no reason to avoid her breasts entirely unless she has indicated that they are temporarily off-limits. And since her body has likely undergone some changes post-pregnancy, be sure to let her know that your reticence to play with her breasts is a reflection of your own uncertainty and not a lack of desire or attraction.

THE MALE ORGASM

The male orgasm is often viewed as simple and straightforward, as it tends to coincide with the observable physiological response of ejaculation. For most men, direct stimulation of the penis takes them over the edge, and they experience a post-climax refractory period that can last from a few minutes to a few days, depending on their age and health. However, men's orgasms can also be varied and complex, and some men reach the heights of pleasure through dreams, prostate stimulation, and B-spot play with or without ejaculation.

During orgasm, the brain and body undergo a powerful eruption of activity as a wave of pleasure spreads across his body. Orgasmic contractions can be felt in his pelvic region, and these are often related to ejaculation. The build-up of pleasant tension is related to the pressure in the prostatic sphincters, and the pulsing sensations are a result of smooth muscle contraction in the testes, seminal vesicles, and prostate. Men usually experience two sets of contractions: The first transports the semen from the testes to the section of urethra below the prostate, and the second involves a release of the sphincter valves to expel the fluid. At the same time, the internal sphincter of the urinary bladder closes to prevent urine from mixing with the semen.

Men's experiences of orgasm vary considerably, and there is no right way to reach climax. You do not have to attempt or embrace every approach to orgasm to have a hot sex life, but broadening your horizons and experimenting with new techniques can be enriching and even transform your relationship with your body.

Although women often talk about their struggles and confusion with orgasm, we often assume that male orgasm is both easy and inevitable. However, for many men, this is simply not the case. Just like women, men can also face challenges in reaching orgasm for a range psychological and physiological reasons. Stress, distraction, alcohol consumption and medication are just a few factors that can impede orgasm.

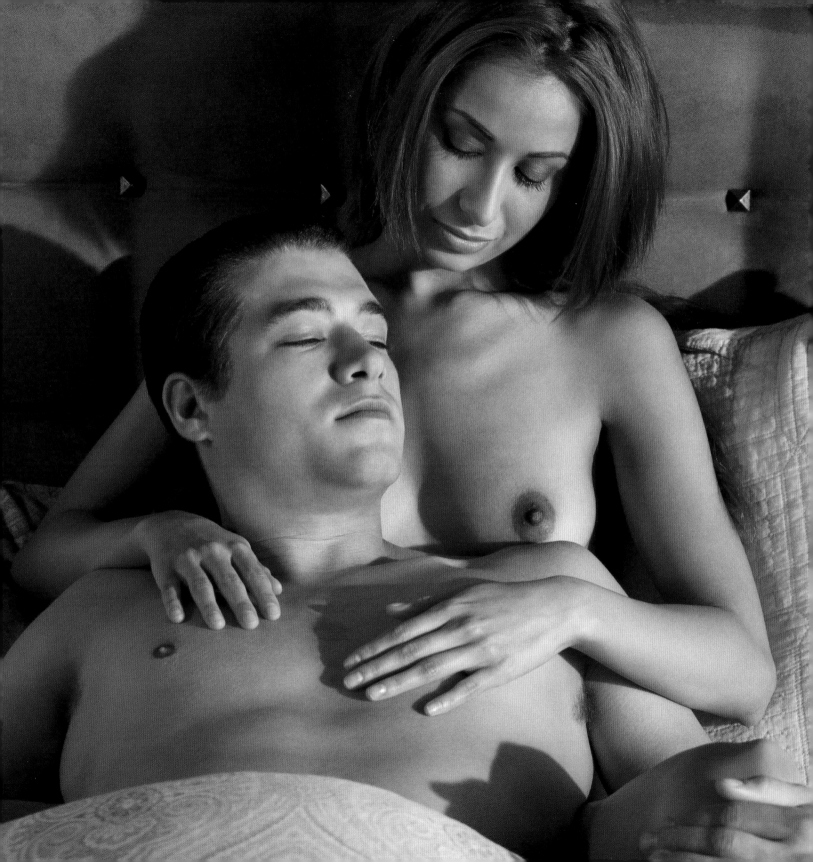

PROSTATE ORGASMS

The prostate gland is located right next to your rectum, just beyond the anal canal. You may have heard that it is located *inside* of your butt, but it's actually a friendly neighbor that rests against the sensitive front of the rectal wall. It is round and somewhat conical in shape and sits in the pelvic cavity between the bladder and the pelvic floor. Responsible for secreting a slightly alkaline fluid that helps to carry and support sperm, for many men, this responsive gland is also a source of undeniable sexual pleasure. Often referred to as the male G-spot, its muscular and glandular tissue surrounds the urethra and swells during arousal like its female counterpart.

To stimulate the prostate gland externally, you can access it through your perineum. Since the sling of muscles along the pelvic floor are relatively thick, you'll need to use considerable pressure to really access this hot spot. Try putting a bit of lube on your hands and pressing your index, middle, and ring fingers in a firm curving motion just in front of the anal opening. Alternatively, you can awaken the prostate using a deep pulsing sensation by slowly pressing and releasing with your flat hand against the full length of the perineum.

Since the prostate sits against the sensitive rectal wall, internal stimulation, or "milking," can be highly pleasurable. To find this hot spot, lie back with your knees pulled into your chest and your legs spread open. Your lover can kneel between your legs and begin with a sensuous external massage to get you primed and then slide a lubed finger into your bum. As she curls it up toward the anterior wall (in the direction of your stomach), she may feel the gland swell with arousal. Try these other tips for internally massaging the prostate:

Curl two fingers up toward the stomach in a slow, "come hither" motion.

Slide a finger back and forth from left to right in a cupping motion.

Pulse two fingers against the prostate gland in rhythm with stroking the penis.

Use a lubed up anal toy like the Aneros to trace slow ovals over the prostate.

Stroke the shaft of his cock while simultaneously curling one finger against his prostate in rhythm with your strokes.

If it is your first time experimenting with anal penetration and internal prostate stimulation, you might feel awkward, tender, or uncomfortable. As you learn to relax your sphincter muscles and become acquainted with your unique reactions, the sensations may become more pleasurable. Many men prefer to have their prostates touched once they're already turned on, as they're more relaxed and less inhibited. For those who enjoy prostate massage, they often describe the erotic sensations

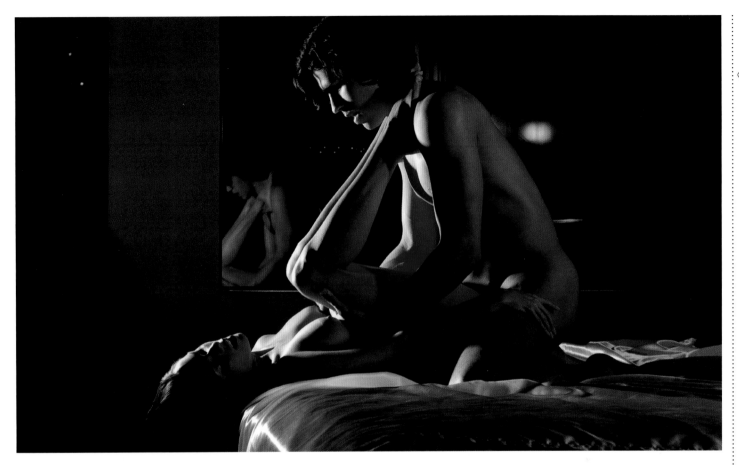

as less location-focused. That is, unlike the penis, which experiences pleasure in a concentrated area, prostate stimulation often results in a more widespread sense of pleasure.

It may take some time to learn to enjoy prostate play, but don't worry if it's not your cup of tea. Just as some women find direct G-spot stimulation irritating or unexciting, some men just don't derive a great deal of pleasure from their prostates. While a little experimentation is almost always a good thing, you don't have to enjoy *every* sexual act imaginable to have a fulfilling sex life.

B-SPOT ORGASMS

The B-spot, or bulb of the penis, is one of the most reactive parts of his body, but it often does not receive the attention it deserves. Located just behind the balls, the bulb or inner penis can be accessed through the perineum. Its hypersensitivity may be related to the fact that it includes extensions of the corpora cavernosa, which fill with blood during erection, and the crura of the penis, which are homologous to the sensitive clitoral legs. The sensitive corpus spongiosum, which surrounds the urethra and forms the very sensitive head of the penis, also extends into this area and is covered by the bulbospongiosus muscle.

We tend to get so hung up on stroking, sucking, and pumping as deeply as possible—stopping at the base of his shaft—yet we neglect the true bedrock of the penis that is located *inside* the body. MRI imaging reveals that the penis assumes a boomerang shape during intercourse and only two-thirds of this powerful organ is located on the outside of his body. The inner portion accounts for the remaining third, taking the full size of an average penis (from inner root to outer tip) to an average of almost nine inches! It seems men have been telling the truth about their penis size all along—so long as we account for the inner portion.

Accessible through the perineum, you can experience B-spot orgasms on their own or in conjunction with intercourse, oral sex, hand jobs, or masturbation. Ask your lover to try these techniques designed to stimulate the B-spot and extend your orgasmic sensations across your pelvic floor:

Expand your blow job to include the bulb. Start with your lips wrapped around his base and two wet fingers pressed into the center point of his perineum. Slide your fingers forward toward his balls, applying firm pressure, and then continue the motion up his shaft, with your lips sucking to the tip. Lower your lips back down and, when they reach the deepest point, slide your finger back to the middle of his perineum as though they are a continuation of your lips. The result should be a more intense blow job that covers his true length inside and out.

Squat over him facing his feet and suck him into your pussy, lowering your lips just beyond his corona. Pop up and down over only his head while you reach down and swirl your thumb around his B-spot in a large circular motion. This move allows you to simultaneously stimulate the outer reaches of the sensitive spongy tissue in his head and bulb.

Kneel on the floor between his legs as he sits on the edge of a couch and press your lips and tongue into his B-spot while you stroke his shaft with your warm, wet, interlaced fingers of both hands. Suck on his perineum with all your might while compressing your tongue against it. The simultaneous pressing (with your tongue) and sucking (with your lips) may sound sloppy, but the sensation will make him tremble with sexual delight.

Combine B-spot stimulation with oral sex *and* prostate play for a triple threat he will never forget: Curl a finger into his butt to massage his prostate while you suck him into your mouth and pulse three fingers against his B-spot.

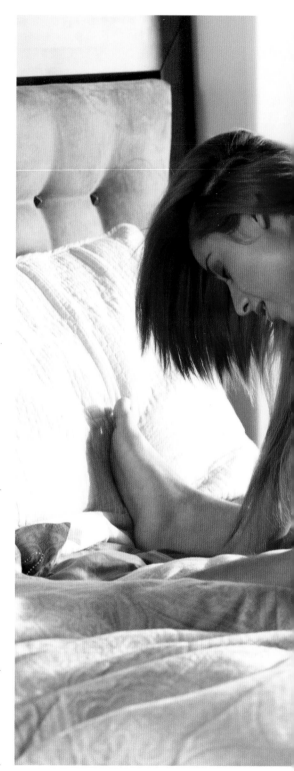

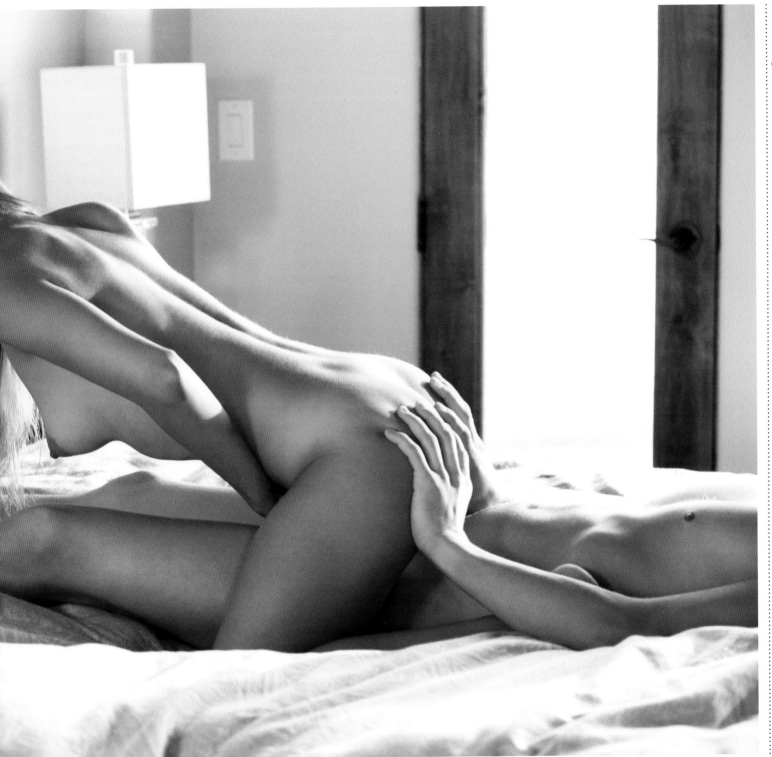

DREAM-GASMS

Nocturnal emissions have long been documented as a way for men to release sexual tension in their sleep. And while women also experience wet dreams, men are twice as likely to have experienced an orgasm in their sleep. Some theorists suggest that sex dreams are a result of heightened dopaminergic systems in conjunction with weakened prefrontal regulatory systems. This theory suggests that our prefrontal cortices help us to control our animalistic and libidinous desires while awake, but as this system gears down during slumber, our reward centers pave the way for hallucinations or dreams. In short, our dreams arise in response to repressed desires.

However, recent research reveals that sex dreams are not particularly common. One study of male college students revealed that men only dream about sex an average of nine times per year. The disparity between incidence of sex dreams versus sex thoughts (even the lowest estimates indicate that men think about sex every day) suggests that dreams cannot solely be extensions of our daily preoccupations and desires. Accordingly, we cannot will ourselves to have sex dreams on demand but can simply embrace them as they arise and take pleasure in the rare occasions in which they result in orgasm.

FOR SEX GEEKS

"Morning wood," also known as nocturnal penile tumescence, is part of your regular sleep pattern, and you likely get erections four to five times per night. When you're awake, the neurotransmitter norepinephrine constricts the blood vessels of the penis to restrict blood flow and prevent erections. But while you sleep, your levels of norepinephrine drop and allow extra blood to flow to the penis, resulting in those friendly boners you wake up with each morning. Scientists believe that these sleep-induced hard-ons actually serve a purpose, as the extra blood flow promotes oxygenation to repair cells, and reflex erections can stop you from wetting the bed.

DRY ORGASMS

While most orgasms are accompanied by ejaculation in men, it is not the fluid expulsion via spinal reflex that produces the wave of pleasure and release of sexual tension associated with orgasm. These gratifying sensations can actually be enjoyed without ejaculation in an experience often referred to as a dry orgasm.

Dry orgasms are sometimes stumbled upon by chance, but some men actually train themselves to enjoy orgasms without ejaculation, as they describe the experience as more intense, and they are able to skip the refractory period and experience multiple orgasms in succession.

As you recall, when male orgasm occurs in conjunction with ejaculation, two set of contractions occur. The first prepares the seminal fluid for expulsion by moving it into the urethral bulb, and the second expels the fluid through the urethral opening. After the first set of contractions, most men reach a point of ejaculator inevitability, as the external sphincter opens and the internal one remains closed to disallow the release of urine and the flow of semen into the bladder. However, dry orgasms can occur between these two sets of orgasmic contractions resulting in *retrograde ejaculation,* in which semen is redirected into the bladder instead of being ejected through the penis.

Anecdotal reports suggest that not all dry orgasms include retrograde ejaculation, but when they do, your urine may appear more cloudy afterward. For men who learn to have dry orgasms at will, experts have not identified any negative side effects. If you'd like to explore the possibility of having dry orgasms, the first step is to tone your pelvic floor muscle. As this area becomes stronger, you can experiment with several approaches to dry orgasm:

Squeeze tightly and flex for a few seconds when you feel orgasm is impending. When you release, you may still experience the wave of orgasmic pleasure and involuntary contractions.

Wait until you reach the point of ejaculatory inevitability to flex your pelvic floor muscle and hold it while breathing deeply until the inclination to ejaculate subsides.

Another option to experiment with dry orgasms involves a slow technique called *edging*. Edging refers to bringing yourself right to the brink of orgasm several times without allowing yourself to go over the edge. Stimulate yourself however you please and stop as soon as you feel as though you are about to climax. Breathe slowly and deeply as you retreat to a less stimulating technique until the urge to ejaculate subsides. Repeat this process several times. With practice, some men find that they eventually experience orgasmic sensations without ejaculation during the retreat period.

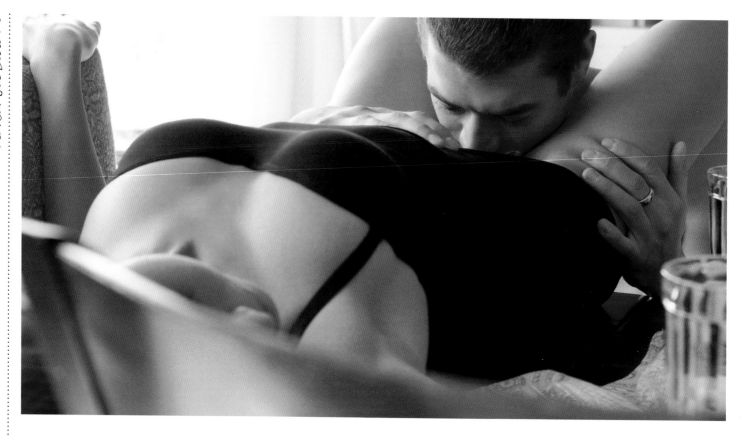

ORGASMS FOR LOVERS

Though our early discoveries of orgasm often arise from solo sex play, exploring our body's climactic reactions with a lover often sparks new pathways to pleasure. As you explore the scintillating world of full-body, multiple, and simultaneous orgasms, you not only expand your sexual horizons but also deepen the erotic connection with your lover and redefine your shared experience of pleasure.

Orgasm may only comprise one part of the sexual experience, but for many people it is the ultimate erotic indulgence. After an orgasm, we often feel relieved, relaxed, and refreshed, so it is no surprise that lovers often feel closer and more in love after an intense climax. These feelings are often associated with experiences of ecstasy and some even describe is as a spiritual experience. Like all genuine sexual experiences, ecstasy is not a goal but a by-product of a powerful connection with oneself or a lover. Those who consider orgasms a source of overwhelming happiness and joy remark that the entire process begins in their minds.

Sexuality specialist Kim Airs describes her experience: "My breath becomes deepened, my mind escapes from my head, my eyes see everything sensual even though they're closed. My skin lightens off the surface where I lie, my pelvis tenses and releases without consciousness, my hands grip anything, even air. The denseness of reality gives way to effortless pleasure that is all mine to keep. Forever."

Full-body orgasms are often compared to out-of-body experiences, as the pleasure overtakes your full form tsunami-style. Our culture's concurrent obsession with and disdain for our genitals makes them both the myopic focus of pleasure and a source of shame. Learning to derive sexual indulgence and satisfaction from our entire body can help us to overcome this contradiction. But full-body orgasms are not just about the *physical* sensations we experience as our arousal peaks; our mind's connection to our sexual enjoyment is of equal importance. Try these tips from erotic massage therapist Sharleen G., who specializes in full-body experiences for couples:

For the receiver:

Wind down and clear your mind by placing your hand on your tummy and taking some deep belly breaths. Focus on the air flow as your tummy rises and drops and allow any intrusive thoughts to float away. Remind yourself that you are deserving of and ready to embrace sexual pleasure.

Roll onto your stomach and allow yourself to soak in all the pleasure your giving lover has to offer.

Breathe deeply, thinking of nothing but the physical sensations in your body and against your skin.

Visualize the pleasure running up your spine, over your shoulders, across your collarbone, down to your fingertips, and throughout your legs.

Allow your natural sounds to emanate uninhibited.

For the giver:

Lower the lights and blindfold your lover, setting your toys, props, and other accouterments within arm's reach.

Move s-l-o-w-l-y as you caress her body. If you think you are moving slowly enough, reduce your speed by half. Do not zone-in on her genitals or other hot areas, as appealing as they may be.

Begin with a gentle scalp massage using the light pads of your fingertips and breathe deeply to encourage your lover's breath.

Slowly work your way down over her neck and shoulder blades, sweeping your palms in light circular motions using a light oil.

Take your time and slide your fingers down her arms trickling your fingernails against the warm path.

Spend at least five minutes caressing, nuzzling, and kissing her hands.

Slide your hands over the small of her back, gradually working your way down over her bum.

Tease her from behind for a brief minute.

Massage her thighs and calves with strong hands and apply more oil liberally.

After at least twenty minutes, roll her over onto her back, ensuring that her blindfold is securely in place

Caress her face, breathe over her lips, swirl your tongue around her ears, and kiss her passionately.

Breathe heavily as you fondle her neck and work your way down her body covering every square inch with your lips, tongue, fingers, and breath.

After another twenty minutes have passed, press your hand into her pubic mound, allowing her to rock against you.

Slide your fingers between her legs or use your tongue to pleasure her. At this point you can climb on top and slide inside if you'd like, but this is completely optional. However you choose to proceed, keep your hands engaged, covering as much of her skin as possible, even as she climaxes.

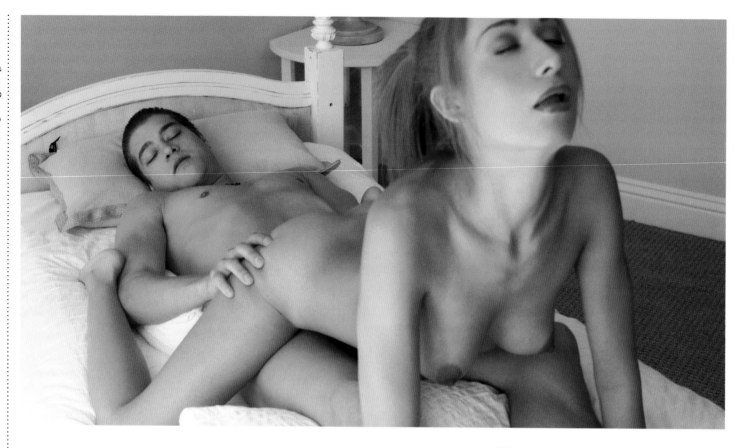

MULTIPLE ORGASMS

Successive orgasms can make great sex even hotter, and both women and men are capable of enjoying multiples.

For Men

Since most men experience a refractory period after they come, dry orgasms may be the best approach to male multiples. Without ejaculation, you can maintain peak arousal levels after orgasm without losing your erection. Learning to have multiple orgasms through dry climaxes takes time, practice, and patience, so do not worry if you are not able to control your physical reactions from the onset. It can take weeks, months, or even longer, and the process should be pleasurable and enlightening as opposed to pressure-laden and frustrating.

Each man's personal journey toward multiple orgasms is unique, so the following suggestions are merely guidelines that you can tweak according to your specific reactions, needs, and experiences:

Do your Kegel exercises and squats regularly (see page 24). Pelvic floor muscle tone is of paramount importance if you want to learn to control ejaculation and intensify orgasms.

Practice controlled breathing in a variety of situations, including nonsexual scenarios. Deep and rhythmic breathing during sex helps to manage our physiological response to sexual stimuli, but most of us hold our breath or take shallow puffs as arousal peaks.

Get to know your body's response to a variety of stimulation techniques beyond simple stroking and thrusting of your penis. Pay specific attention to the high point of arousal just before orgasm so that you can identify how your mind, body, genitals, and skin react.

When you reach the highest point of the plateau stage just before orgasm, stop what you're doing and stay still. Squeeze your pelvic floor muscle while pressing firmly into the area of your perineum just in front of your anus to stimulate your prostate. Breathe deeply and allow the prostatic contractions and orgasmic sensations to travel throughout your body.

When your orgasmic contractions cease, release your pelvic floor muscle and take a few deep breaths before resuming stimulation.

For Women

Some women have several orgasms in a row without reverting to the early stages of sexual arousal, and others have a series of less intense orgasms culminating in a more powerful climax. Some have orgasms that are considerably spaced out, and others report that they enjoy alternating between orgasms generated from clitoral stroking and those that originate from G-spot pressure. There is no comprehensive formula to enjoying multiples, but these approaches will enhance your sexual experience regardless of how many times you climax:

After orgasm, your clitoris can become hypersensitive, so most women avoid direct stimulation. However, some women say that if you push through and embrace the seemingly unbearable overstimulation, your pleasure will build back up quickly, resulting in a subsequent orgasm.

As you orgasm, you experience muscular contractions accompanied by heightened sensation throughout your body. Pulse your hand against your entire vulva, G-spot, or clitoral head (depending on your primary source of pleasure) in between each contraction and squeeze your thighs together to prolong the contractions and carry you to the next wave of orgasmic bliss.

When you reach orgasm, breathe as slowly and deeply as possible while contracting your pelvic floor muscle. Some women report that this technique makes the orgasmic sensations last longer.

Change up your technique after orgasm. If your first orgasm occurs as a result of clitoral stimulation, give this area a break and switch to G-Spot, breast, or anal play. Since you'll already be highly aroused, you don't have to start from scratch and can experience successive orgasms that feel entirely different than those that preceded them.

DR. JESS SAYS . . .

If you want to experiment with multiple orgasms, consider wearing a cock ring (page 185) to see if it helps you to maintain greater ejaculatory control. While some men find that contraction of their pelvic floor muscle staves off orgasm, others experience the opposite and find that it makes them come even harder. This contradictory information may seem confusing, but it is simply a reminder that there is no perfect technique that produces a universal outcome when it comes to sex.

SIMULTANEOUS ORGASMS

Coming together can be an intimate and intense bonding experience that many couples stumble upon by chance. Though often associated with feelings of closeness, reaching orgasm at the same time is not a particularly common occurrence. This is because each of our bodies responds at a different pace, making it impossible to be consistently in synch with a lover. Just as you cannot possibly digest food, pump blood, or lose weight at the same rate as your partner, you also cannot expect your orgasmic responses to line up perfectly each and every time.

Despite the fact that simultaneous orgasms don't often occur naturally, there are some techniques you can employ to get your arousal in synch and increase your chances of reaching climax around the same time:

Breathe in rhythm with one another to deepen your connection and synchronize the movements of your bodies.

Learn to control your sexual response. If you tend to reach orgasm before your partner, slow your response through breath work, pelvic floor squeezes, positional changes, or varied techniques. For example, men who come more quickly might benefit from a shallow-penetration position like the T-Bone (see page 96), whereas women who orgasm with great speed might be able to slow things down by switching from direct clitoral stimulation to vaginal penetration.

Slow down! Sex is not a race, but many of us treat orgasms as though they are the ultimate finish line. Take your time to enjoy the journey.

Masturbate! Self-pleasure before a sex session can help you to control your orgasmic response, allowing a partner who moves at a more leisurely pace to catch up.

Make eye contact. Gazing in to your lover's eyes not only deepens the intimate connection, but it can also help you to gauge when orgasm is impending.

Talk to one another. Let your lover know if you're close to orgasm with some practical dirty talk: "I'm going to come soon," "I'm getting close," or "Get ready for my come!"

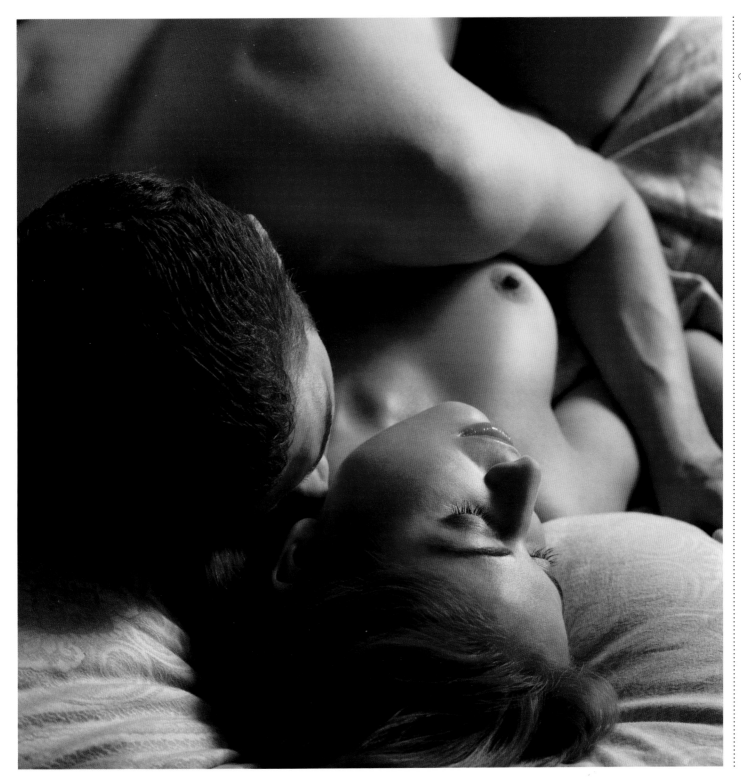

MORE-GASMS

DELAYED GRATIFICATION

Delaying gratification can have a tremendous impact on sexual response as the backlog of tension results in powerful yearning, leading to stronger orgasms. You can use delayed gratification to tempt your lover all week long or tease and tantalize his body during a single sex session to build orgasmic energy to new highs.

For example, take a sex hiatus and agree to no sexual touch for a full week. Wear sexy clothes, bend over provocatively, and tease in every way possible so that you are both aching to tear one another's clothes off. When you finally give in, the sexual tension will create attraction, desire, and arousal levels similar to those you experienced when you first met. You may also want to deprive your lover of kissing for a brief time or hide her favorite vibrator and tease her to the brink of orgasm several times before finishing her off. These strategies also pair well with dominant/submissive interactions, as you might use delayed gratification as a means of control and dominance.

The power of delayed gratification is related to greater self-regulation, so if your lover is impatient, remind her that the benefits of training yourself to control impulsive behavior are many. Not only is it connected to social competence and psychological well-being but also to improved health and professional success. Interestingly, studies suggest that women are more likely to delay rewards than men, but you might want to turn this into a playful competition and see who can hold out longer.

FAKING IT

Faking orgasms is a common sexual practice, with most women (and some men) putting on Oscar-worthy performances at some point in their lives. And apparently male partners are none the wiser. The National Survey of Sexual Health and Behavior found that 85 percent of men believed that their female partners achieved orgasm during their last sex session. But only 64 percent of women reported that they had. Talk about a gender gap.

Our reasons for faking it vary from the obvious well-intentioned ego-stroking to the utilitarian need to "get it over with already." However, faking it is bad education and reinforces less-than-stellar approaches to pleasure. Sex is supposed to be one of those things you do because it *feels* good—not because you feel pressure to do

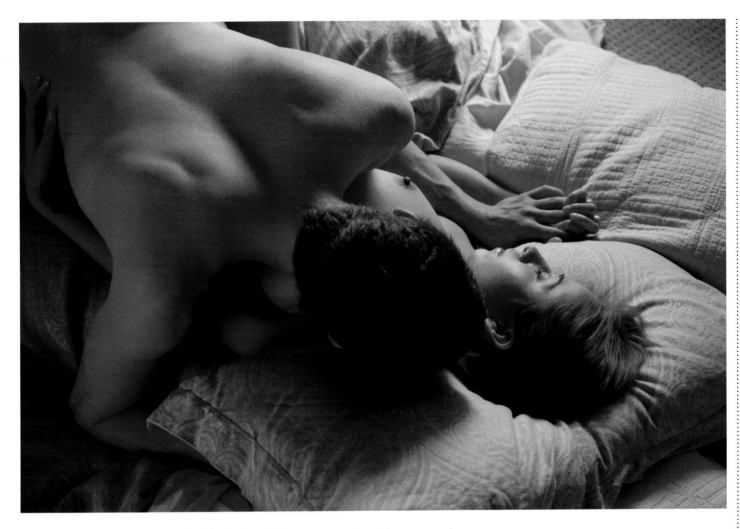

so. The flip side is that your partner shouldn't feel pressure to perform or "give" you an orgasm. If you pretend to like something that doesn't really tickle your fancy, you're ultimately leading your partner down the wrong path, and chances are you will get a whole lot more of what you don't like in the future.

Offering *some* positive reinforcement and elements of exaggeration can amp up your bedroom routine, but you certainly do not want to do so at the expense of your own pleasure. So the next time you're getting down and not genuinely feeling the vibe, instead of inflating your dramatic performance, take your partner by the hand (or penis or mouth) and offer some guidance. You don't need to kill the moment altogether or complain, "This isn't doing it for me," but offer good-natured reminders or suggestions that enhance the mood: "I love when you use your hands like that" or "I really like when you lick me right there!"

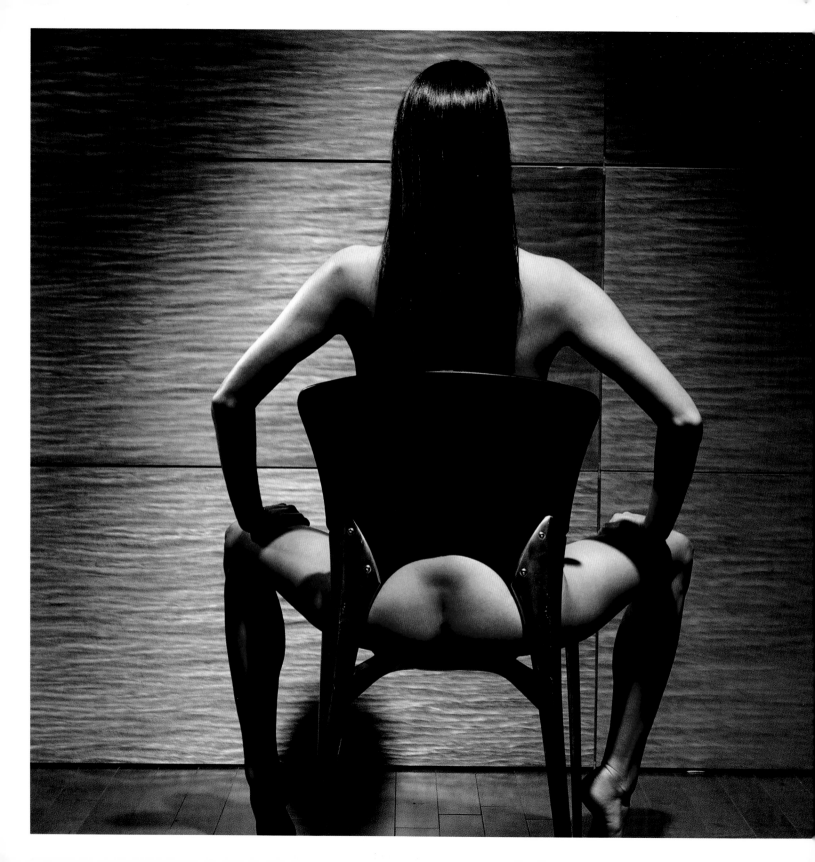

06 *Anal Play*

Your bum is one of the most responsive erogenous zones on your body, so exploring its pleasure potential is a no-brainer. Not only is the anus rich in super-sensitive nerve endings, but it is actually anatomically configured for mind-blowing orgasms for both men and women: The male G-spot, also known as the prostate, and the female cul-de-sac, that sexy region on the lower vaginal wall, can be stimulated through the back door.

ANAL SEX TIPS

Despite the climax-centered design of the bum, anal sex continues to retain its taboo status…at least in theory. In reality, anal sex is quite common. Research suggests that nearly half of men and women have engaged in anal intercourse, and orgasm rates are actually higher for women who include anal play in their erotic repertoire. That's right! According to the National Survey of Sexual Health and Behavior conducted by the Center for Sexual Health Promotion at Indiana University in Bloomington, among women who had anal sex during their last encounter, 94 percent had an orgasm versus only 84 percent of those who received oral and 65 percent of those who had vaginal intercourse.

Couple the powerful potential for orgasm with the thrill of defying one of the most intense and enduring sexual taboos, and you have the perfect recipe for spicing up your sex life! But since the tissue and nerve endings of the anal area are so sensitive, it is essential to follow some basic guidelines to make sure your experience is as hot as possible.

Become acquainted with your bum. Your ass is a thing of wonder, but since you probably don't know this nether region like the back of our hand, you'll want to do some exploring before you venture into the exciting land of anal play.

On the outside, you have a highly responsive pucker (aka bum hole/anus) that is rich in nerve endings and responsive to light touch. For some people, this is where anal sex begins and ends. There is nothing in the rule book that says you must include penetration in your anal sex practice. A good exercise for newbies to build trust and become familiar with new sensations is to enjoy anal play (licking, sucking, massaging, kissing, etc.) with the promise of no penetration.

If you do decide to venture inside, you'll enter the anal canal, which is less than a few inches long and rich in highly responsive nerve endings. Comprised of soft tissue folds, this area has a good capacity for expansion and is sensitive to touch, pressure, and temperature.

Inside, you'll find two sphincter muscles, which are ring-like oval structures that help to hold the canal in shape. The next time you're in the shower and feeling relaxed, gently slide a lubed finger inside to get to know your sphincter muscles. You don't have to reach great depths to find them. You'll feel the external sphincter, which you can contract and release at will (the way you might flex and relax your biceps) less than an inch beyond the opening. The internal sphincter is just a little deeper, but because this smooth muscle ring is controlled by the autonomic nervous system (which manages automatic bodily functions like heartbeat and perspiration), it remains in a state of contraction. You can't exercise complete control over your internal sphincter, but just as you can slow your heart rate through breathing and mindfulness, so too can you help relax this sensitive muscle through relaxation and deep breaths.

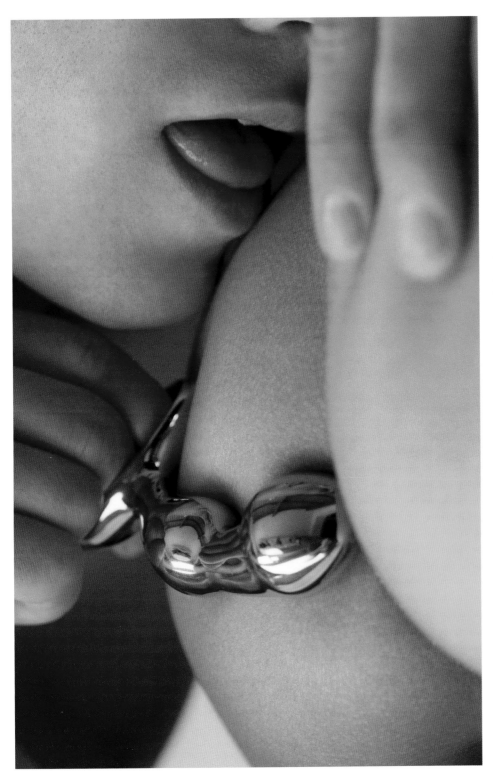

Beyond the anal canal lies the rectum, which comprises the lower section of the large intestine. This section curves laterally (from side to side) as well as from front-to-back several times, and it is wider that the anal canal. Made up of mucous membrane, this deeper zone may be less responsive to light touch but more reactive to pressure.

DIY. As a general rule, the best way to venture into unchartered sexual territory is to experiment on your own before bringing a partner into the equation. This is because solo sex helps to detract from performance pressure, and when we're alone we often allow our natural bodily responses to flow more freely. So if you're curious about butt play, but don't know where to start, begin by playing with your own bum first to get an idea of how it might feel with a partner.

Don't have a one-track mind. Don't get hung up exclusively on the butt! We all have a tendency to get fixated on a body part or sex act when we're excited, nervous, or trying something out for the first time. But there is no reason that you have to focus *exclusively* on the bum during anal play. Double your pleasure and use a spare hand to rub her clitoris or stroke his cock to produce arousal patterns with which your brain and body are already familiar.

Proceed gradually. Anal sex should not be painful, so proceeding gradually in terms of speed, depth, and the size of inserted object is of paramount importance. Take time to deepen your breathing and begin with a very small object like your pinky finger before increasing the size gradually. If you decide that anal penetration is something you enjoy, you may want to invest in an anal trainer kit, which includes various sizes of toys and plugs with flared bases for safety. Start with the smallest one, holding it completely still at first and notice the way your body responds as you allow your muscles to relax around its girth. Work your way up slowly—over days, weeks, or even months—knowing that sex is not a race to the finish line and incremental experimentation can lead to mind-blowing results.

Shelve penetration until you're highly aroused. It is often a good idea to hold off on penetration until you're decidedly excited, as arousal can help you to relax and have a palliative effect on your body. Get yourself all riled up using the techniques and body parts you normally play with before introducing new moves or exploring new regions of the body. And once you've incorporated butt-play into the mix, don't abandon your tried-and-true routines entirely. Instead, start by making backdoor pleasure an addendum to your regular repertoire as opposed to an alternative.

Eat fiber! The link between diet and sexual satisfaction cannot be overstated—especially when it comes to anal sex. If you don't have enough fiber in your diet, it can force you to push harder when using the bathroom resulting in irritation, discomfort, and muscle strain.

FAQ: I'VE TRIED ANAL BEFORE, BUT IT HURT, SO I'M THINKING OF TRYING A NUMBING CREAM. DO THEY WORK, AND ARE THEY SAFE?

There are many numbing creams and lubes on the market designed to help "ease" penetration through the use of a topical anesthetic. Though these creams may not be dangerous in terms of content alone, their desensitizing effect can increase your risk of injury during anal play. The anus is not only sensitive but also thin-skinned and prone to small tears that increase the risk of infection. By temporarily numbing your butt (and by extension, your partner's penis during anal intercourse), you are not only less likely to stop if you experience a small tear but also more likely to experience pain once the cream's effects wear off.

A more pleasurable and safer alternative to numbing creams involves more foreplay, lots of lube, and high levels of relaxation prior to penetration.

SEX TIP FROM THE PROS

Bring yourself to orgasm before experimenting with anal penetration so that your pelvic floor slips into a state of relaxation. Your body is most responsive to pleasure and primed for arousal when your endorphin and oxytocin levels are elevated post-orgasm.

FINGER AND TONGUE PLAY

When most of us think of anal sex, we assume that it includes a penis sliding in and out of the butt. But the reality is that the hottest and most practiced anal techniques often preclude insertion or involve gentle, shallow penetration with smaller objects.

Since the bulk of your most responsive nerve endings are located near the entrance of the ass, your dexterous fingers and nimble tongue make the perfect pleasure tools. Fingering the bum is the ideal way to learn more about your own response to anal pleasure, and rimming/analingus (licking, kissing, and sucking the butt) allows you to experiment with a softer side of anal play. As you take these simple techniques for a backroads test-drive, ask your lover for feedback to guide you in exploring new approaches to pleasure.

BREATHE IT IN

Use nothing but your heavy breath to prime your lover's ass for a night of lovin'! Get as close as you can to her skin without touching her and breathe warm kisses on her lower back, between her butt cheeks, over her pucker, and around her perineum. Alternate between breath kisses and deep, pleasurable inhales as you tell her how much you love it.

A LOTTA HOT AIR

Lick your lips and open them wide as you breathe warm air over your lover's pucker. Gently flatten your tongue against the opening and then purse your lips to breathe cooler air over the soft, wet spot you've created.

DEAR DAISY

Use the soft pad of your thumb (slathered in lube) to trace petals around his pucker as you breathe gently over the wet spot.

EAT YOUR HEART OUT

Use your hands to pry open your lover's supple butt cheeks and dive in with your lips, nose, and tongue. Slurp, kiss, lick, twirl, and suck away as though you're diving face-first into a bowl of freshly whipped cream.

SLIP 'N' SLIDE

Slather your hand in lube and slide it in a very gentle karate chop–style motion between your honey's butt cheeks starting at the very top. Once she is fully relaxed, slither your tongue up and down from the tip of her upper cheeks down to her bum hole.

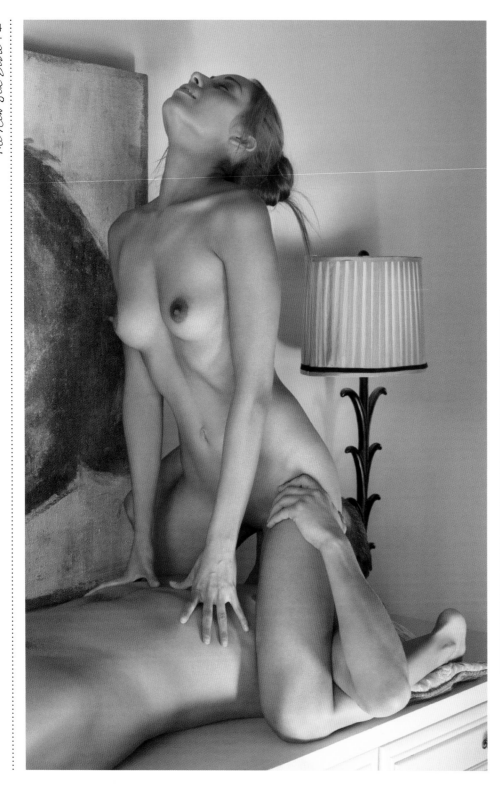

FAQ: I'M TOTALLY STRAIGHT, BUT MY WIFE WANTS TO TRY PUTTING SOMETHING IN MY ASS. I KNOW IT DOESN'T MAKE ME GAY, BUT I CAN'T SEEM TO GET OVER THE IDEA THAT STRAIGHT GUYS DON'T DO IT.

The exclusive association between butt play and gay men is long established, yet erroneous and highly limiting. Many people, including straight men and women, enjoy anal penetration, and the range of sexual activities that include the butt is vast. If you want to let her experiment with butt play, and you enjoy it, this is not an indication that you're gay. Period.

THE REACH AROUND

While you're performing oral sex on your lover, reach around with a wet hand and circle your fingers around his butt hole. Press gently against the opening and gradually slide the tip of your finger inside as you continue to suck away. Hold your finger perfectly still at first and allow him to "suck" it in farther using his sphincter muscles should he so choose. If he can handle a little more action, gently rotate your finger from your wrist as you slide it in just a little deeper.

THE REVERSE REACH

Twirl your tongue around her pucker and gently slide the tip in and out while you reach your flat hand around to stroke her entire vulva to double the pleasure. As you slide your tongue in and out, try rolling it into a tube or curling it gently between her cheeks.

SIT ON MY FACE

Lie on your back with your tongue sticking straight out and have your lover kneel over your face as she sits atop your face and guides your tongue's direction, pressure, and depth. This is the perfect move for newbies, as it allows the receptive partner to maintain total control.

Remember that you don't have to stay exclusively focused on the butt for this move; you can slide back and forth to kiss, lick, and suck her wet lips or his sensitive balls.

BUTT PLUG BONUS

Slide a butt plug in her ass and twirl it around as you swipe a soft tongue all around her hot pussy. Ask her to submit to your control over her front side while allowing her to take the reins of control in the rear.

TAWDRY TRACE

Trace a slow, sensuous line from the center of your lover's spine right down to his pucker and then point your tongue tightly to slide it inside. Alternatively, you can tease him to the heights of desire by slowly working your tongue down his spine.

BUTT SCREW

Cross your ring and middle finger, slather them in lube and slide them into your lover's already primed pucker with your palm facing down. As you pull out, rotate your palm upward and repeat, allowing your partner's hip movements to guide you into a sensual rhythm.

LIP SMACKER

Use two fingers to gently tap her pucker, gradually increasing the intensity and alternating between "smacks" and slurpy wet lip kisses.

TONGUE TWISTER

Hold his ass cheeks open with your hands and slide your tongue inside. Once you're as deep as you can reach, twirl your tongue in a circular fashion to titillate the sensitive nerve endings inside the canal.

SLURPEE

Press your lips around her bum hole in a wide open oval and thrust your tongue flat against it. Slurp away as though you're sucking on a bottle, allowing your natural sounds to emanate freely.

"For men, there is nothing more disheartening than when you have to explain that you are having a good time—even if your soft penis seems to indicate otherwise! I was in a new and very adventurous relationship. I told her that I love having my ass played with so she began massaging my anus. I was loving it, especially when she inserted her finger. At one point she stopped and asked, "Am I doing it wrong?" I tried to assure her that she was doing quite well, but she looked concerned and asked, "Then why aren't you hard anymore?" I explained that usually happens when you touch a guy's ass. So many other fantastic sensations take over!"

—Jon, 39

PROSTATE PLAY

The prostate, which can be stimulated through the perineum or the inside of his butt, is a remarkable source of pleasure. Many men who have experienced prostate pleasure will tell you that, on its own or in conjunction with vaginal intercourse, anal intercourse, oral sex, and manual play, they blow penile orgasms out of the water.

But don't expect a rock-hard erection every time. Sometimes prostate play results in a hard-on and other times the penis is flaccid or only partially erect, despite the mind-numbing pleasure he experiences during it.

Charlie Glickman, Ph.D., sex coach and author of *The Ultimate Guide to Prostate Pleasure*, explains that one possible reason is that "relaxing the pelvic muscles enough to allow penetration means that less blood is trapped in the penis. Another is that some guys need direct stimulation to stay erect. And if he's feeling any concerns or worries about anal penetration, the stress can short-circuit the erection process. If his toes are curling and he's having a great time, there's no reason to get worked up over whether he has an erection."

For some amazing prostate massage techniques, refer back to Prostate Orgasms on page 144.

Dr. Glickman notes that it's fairly common for guys to ejaculate more semen from a prostate massage, "since you're squeezing more fluid out of the gland. In fact, you might end up with more pre-cum along the way." He suggests putting your man on his hands and knees "for a gravity assist" and setting a towel under him because "the wet spot will be huge!"

PERFECT POSITIONS FOR ANAL

If you're ready to move on to anal intercourse, finding the right positions to maximize both comfort and pleasure is of paramount importance. The following positions are designed with both of your needs in mind, so take them for a test drive and see which ones tickle your fancy. As mentioned, take your time with foreplay, and be generous with the lube before beginning any anal play.

REVERSE COWGIRL

This is the ideal lady-on-top position for the domme who loves to maintain control. Ideal for anal intercourse, the Reverse Cowgirl lets her determine the depth of penetration, angle of entry, and speed of the ride while he sits back and enjoys the view.

Take Position

He lies on his back and she kneels over his pelvic region facing his feet.

She slathers his cock with lube before sucking him into her tight butt using her hand for guidance.

He places his hands on her plump butt cheeks to provide extra support as needed.

She can slide up and down over the head of his cock, rock back and forth to massage her inner walls, or pop her butt backward in a circular motion to stroke his shaft.

SEX TIPS FROM THE PROS

If she doesn't like deep penetration, but he desires more stimulation against the base of his shaft, she can reach backward with a warm, wet hand to grasp the lower half of his cock. Her hand becomes an extension of her butt while providing a physical buffer to ensure only shallow penetration.

SLITHERING SNAKE

This more advanced anal sex position has everything you need for coupled orgasms, providing deep penetration and thrusting for him and dual stimulation of the cul-de-sac and clitoris for her.

To limit the depth of penetration while maintaining the excitement of deep thrusting movements, consider wearing a Not-So-Deep Donut ring (or two), which sits on the base of his penis.

Take Position

She lies on her stomach with her legs slightly apart and her hands beneath her pubic mound.

He straddles her on his knees and slides in from behind as she lifts her hips to facilitate entry.

As he thrusts, he leans forward supporting himself with his hands on either side of her shoulders.

She allows the weight of her body (and his) to press into her fingers at the top of her pubic mound. As he thrusts, she pulls up on her mound to provide intense stroking to the shaft and head of her clitoris.

SEX TIPS FROM THE PROS

Add vibrations into the mix with the Slithering Snake, and the sensory overload will launch her pleasure to new heights. Choose a flat vibrator like the We-Vibe Touch and slide it beneath her clitoris, allowing the weight of your bodies to enhance the sensations.

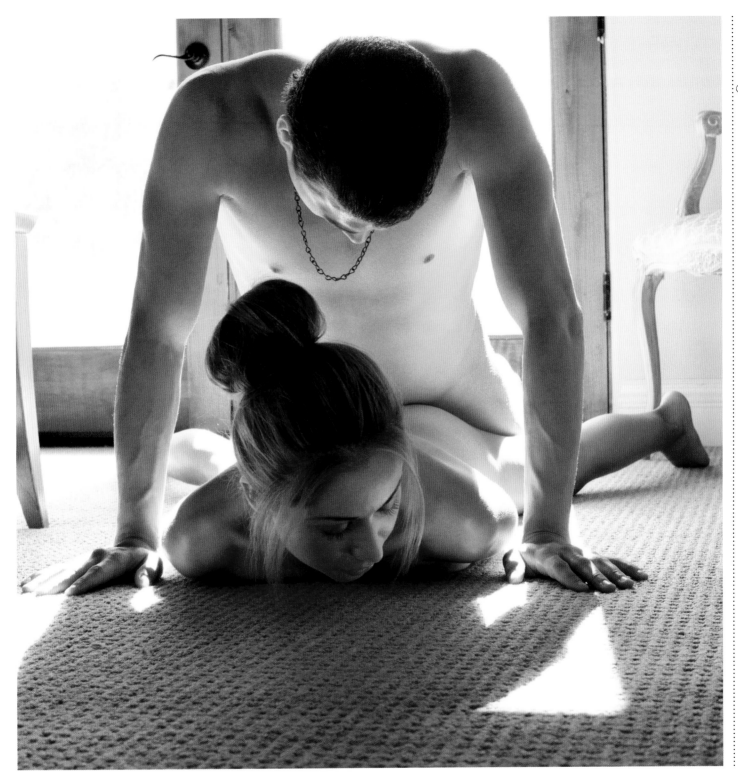

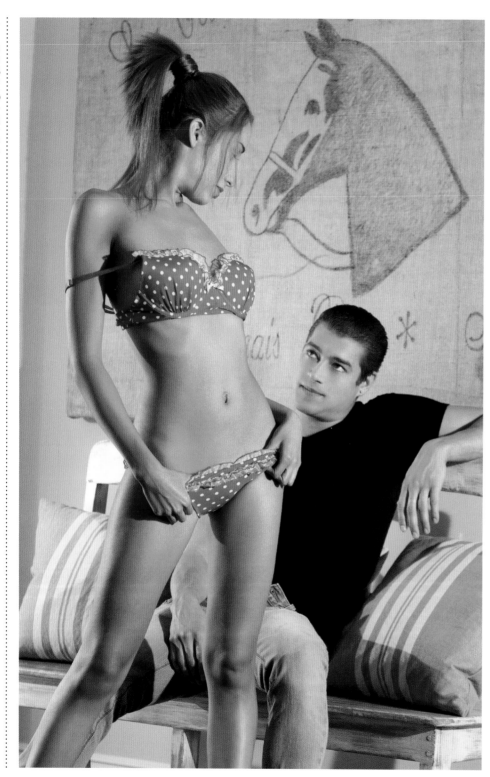

SEX TIPS FROM THE PROS

If you've ever fantasized about double penetration, the Modified Doggie can help bring that fantasy to life. In this position, he can reach around and slide a finger or toy into her pussy while she continues to wrap her sweet pucker around his cock. Alternatively, she can reach down and finger herself in tempo with her own thrusting.

To ensure that the pressure of her tight pucker doesn't cause him any pain or discomfort, he can hold his own cock at the base to make sure that it slides inside of her and doesn't receive any direct impact from her tailbone.

MODIFIED DOGGIE

In the traditional doggie-style position, she rests on her hands and knees while he enters from behind in a kneeling position. While this creates a hot setup for vaginal sex, the modified doggie is ideal for anal, as it gives the receptive partner more control, facilitates greater intimacy, and frees up your hands to fondle other hot spots while you rock together in perfect rhythm.

Take Position

She assumes a kneeling position with her butt cheeks on her heels and her knees spread wide open. She places her hands on her knees or the bed for support.

He assumes the same position behind her and adjusts his height so that the head of his cock rests below her bum.

He remains static as she lowers herself onto his head and takes a few deep breaths before sliding farther down his shaft.

She drives her ass and hips up and down at her own pace as he reaches around to fondle her tits or rub her clit.

REAR-VIEW LAP DANCE

If you've ever been to a strip club (or seen one in a movie), you know that the dancers harness their power by teasing, tantalizing...and saving the best for last. The Rear-View Lap Dance position allows her to exercise complete control as she works him into a desperate sexual frenzy.

Take Position

He sits on an armless chair as she sashays around him wearing nothing but a bra, panties, and heels.

She teasingly unclasps her bra from behind but leaves the straps on so that the cups reveal only the soft mounds peeking out from below.

She demands that he peel off her panties and helps him by lifting one foot through the loop and leaving the panties wrapped around her other ankle.

With her back to him, she gradually lowers herself down over his rock-hard cock, teasing his head with her wet pucker.

She reaches behind and wraps her fingers around his shaft ever so slowly while gradually guiding his head into her warm, tight ass.

After a few pumps at a very shallow depth, she slides a little deeper and repeats until she feels totally relaxed encompassing his entire length.

DR. JESS SAYS . . .

You can experiment with variations of the Rear-View Lap Dance position to add spice and variety to your routine: She can bend over and grab her ankles to change the angle and alter the sensations for both partners, or she can turn around and sit on his lap in a face-to-face position.

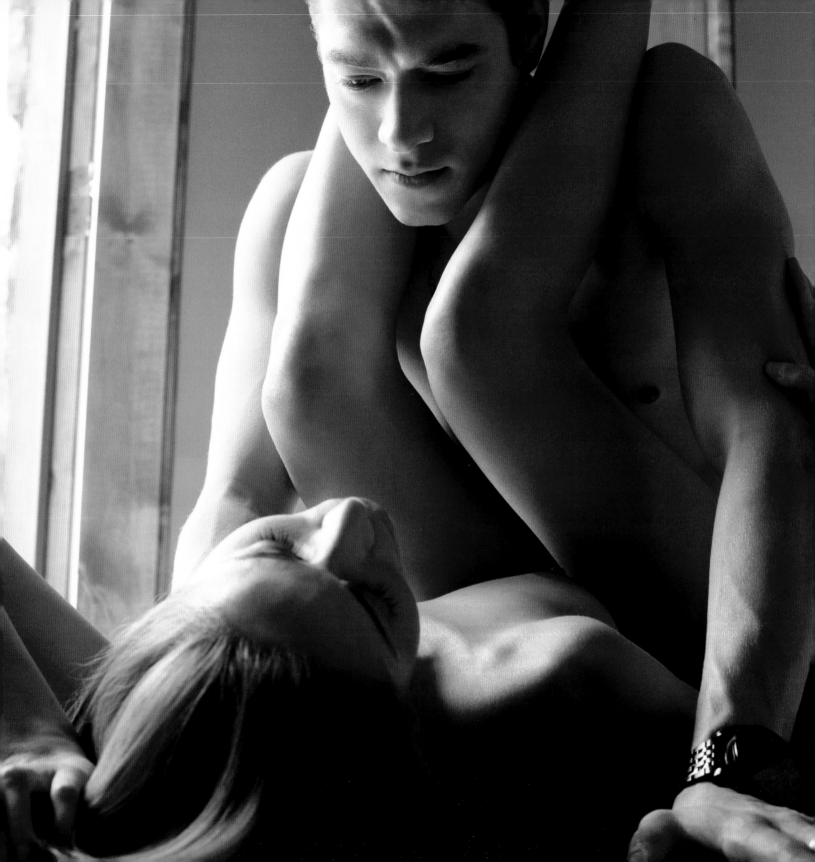

If deep penetration isn't your cup of tea, she can limit his depth by pressing the soles of her feet into his chest to keep him at bay. Discuss your roles and boundaries in advance, and you can pair her resistance with his forcefulness to act out a kinky scene of playing hard-to-get.

TABLE TOP

The Table Top position allows for deep penetration and the added intensity of eye contact during an intimate yet taboo act. It is ideal for those who are more experienced with anal intercourse, as it requires a bit of flexibility and a good deal of trust between partners.

Take Position

She lies on her back on a hip-height table or bed with her butt right on the edge and her legs hanging off the side.

He stands on the floor in front of her and lifts her legs, allowing her feet to rest on his shoulders.

He slides in and pumps away, pressing her legs toward her head to increase the depth of penetration.

SQUATTER

The Squatter position may be a great calorie-burner, but its appeal is really in its versatility. Because the inner butt doesn't run in a perfectly straight line, anal sex requires some flexibility and experimentation. This position is ideal for discovering exactly which angles, movements, and depth work for you.

Take Position

He lies flat on his back with his arms away from his sides.

She squats on her feet over his groin and lowers herself onto his cock.

FAQ: HOW DO I GET OVER THE IDEA THAT ANAL SEX IS DIRTY?

Rest assured that anal play is only dirty in the hottest sense of the word. Regular hygiene and grooming routines (e.g., daily showers or baths) keep the anus clean. Having said that, the bum is a passageway for feces, so having a shower before anal play and sliding a finger up your bum to clean it out or double check will help to put you at ease.

Dr. Glickman notes that there is still some risk for sexually transmitted infections, as well as GI bugs like giardia. "Use a safer sex barrier, like plastic wrap or a dental dam. Put some lube on the side that will be in contact with your partner and hold the barrier in place with your hands."

NOT-SO-SWEET SPOONS

Spooning is the perfect position for lovers! As you press the full length of your bodies into one another, the physical contact causes a spike in oxytocin, which promotes bonding, intimacy, and relaxation. Since this rear-entry position limits his depth of penetration, it is ideal for men with larger penises.

The Not-So-Sweet Spoons position can take on a life of its own depending on your mood. He can gently caress her breasts from behind while she tilts back to kiss his neck, or he can pull her hair and spank her ass a little to showcase his rougher side.

Take Position

She lies on her side and he lies behind her in the same position with his chest pressed against her back.

He lifts her upper leg up slightly and slides inside.

She wraps her upper leg back over his legs and reaches down to fondle herself.

She can control the pace and depth by popping her hips back into him, or she can lie still and hand over the reins of control.

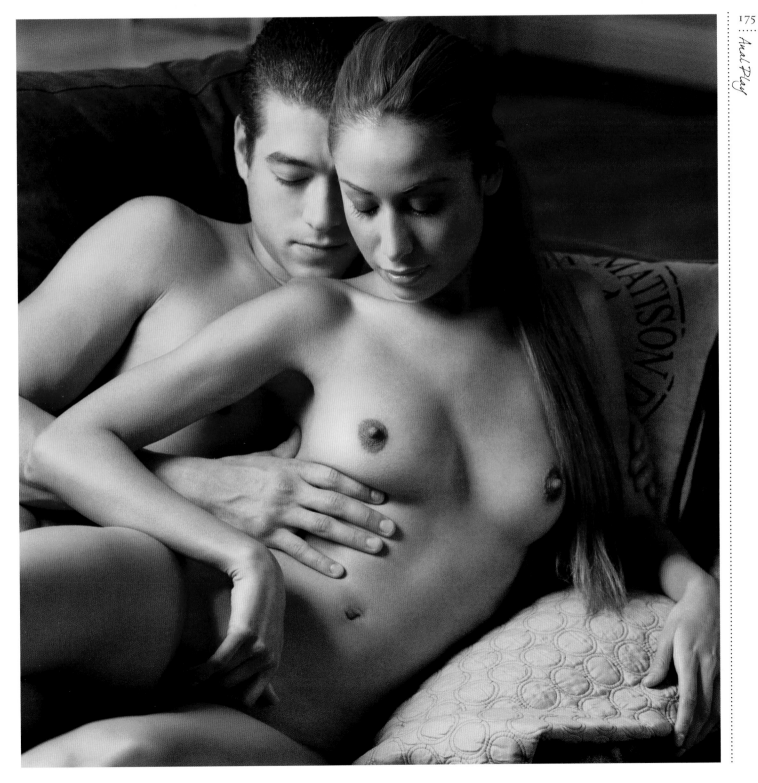

OVERCOMING ANAL SEX HICCUPS

As hot as anal sex can be, it is not uncommon for newbies and experts alike to run into a few obstacles along the way. From the physical to the psychological, most of these challenges can be successfully managed with a little patience, relaxation, and a few practical additions to your sexual routine.

If you can't get it in the hole . . . Fret not! Take a few slow, deep breaths and play with yourself or your lover in a way that is more familiar and relaxing. When you're nervous, anxious, or uncomfortable, your muscles contract, making penetration next to impossible.

Once you're a bit more relaxed and aroused, use your hands to spread your butt cheeks and add some extra lube to your pucker. Push outward as though you're trying to go to the bathroom as you slide a small object (like a finger or the tip of a butt plug) inside. It might seem counterintuitive, but as you bear down with your anal muscles, you'll actually facilitate entry as your muscles expand to open your pucker around the inserted object.

If you experience pain or discomfort with penetration . . . Stop what you're doing, slow down, change angles, or reduce the depth of penetration. Anal sex shouldn't hurt. You may need to add more lube or downgrade to a smaller object. Try inserting a lubed finger inside and holding it perfectly still. Breathe deeply as you become familiar with the sensations of your sphincter muscles. If your internal sphincter is still tightly contracted, take your time breathing to allow it to relax. It may take several sessions over the course of many weeks to relax it to the point of pleasure.

Don't be discouraged if it takes some time to become accustomed to anal play. Rushing into it can cause trauma and is probably the most common rookie mistake. You have lots of body parts from which you can derive sensational pleasure, and your anus isn't going anywhere! If not tonight, then perhaps tomorrow, next week, or next month.

If you feel like you have to go to the bathroom (receptive partner) . . . This is a common sensation, particularly for anal sex novices, since anal sex can awaken the same nerve endings that are impacted when you use the bathroom. Chances are, you don't actually have to go, but to reassure yourself, you can always take a break or empty your bowels and shower before you get down to business.

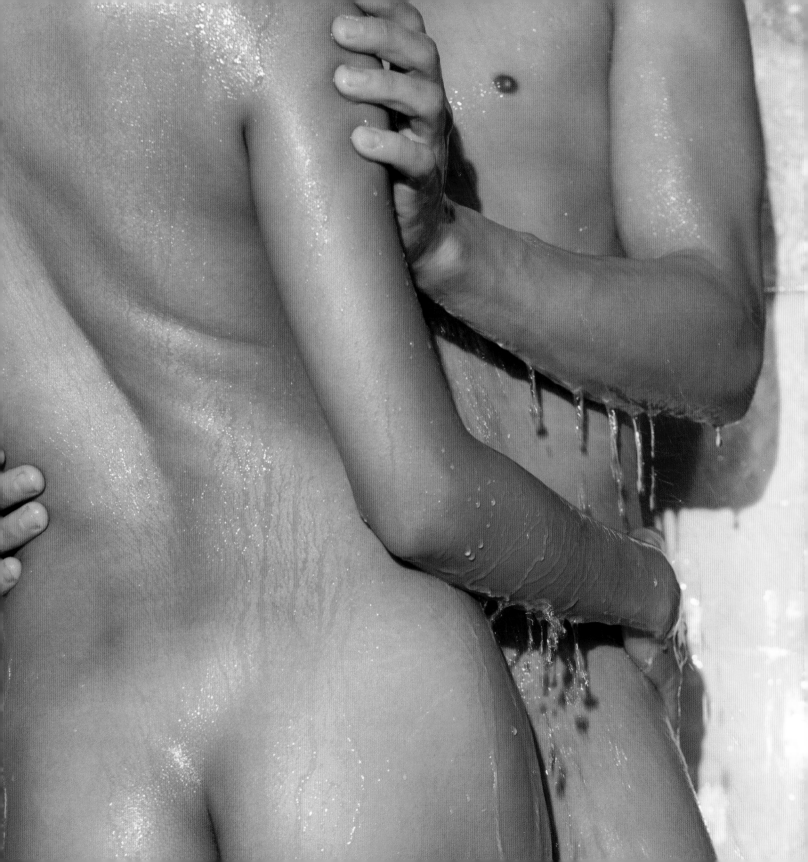

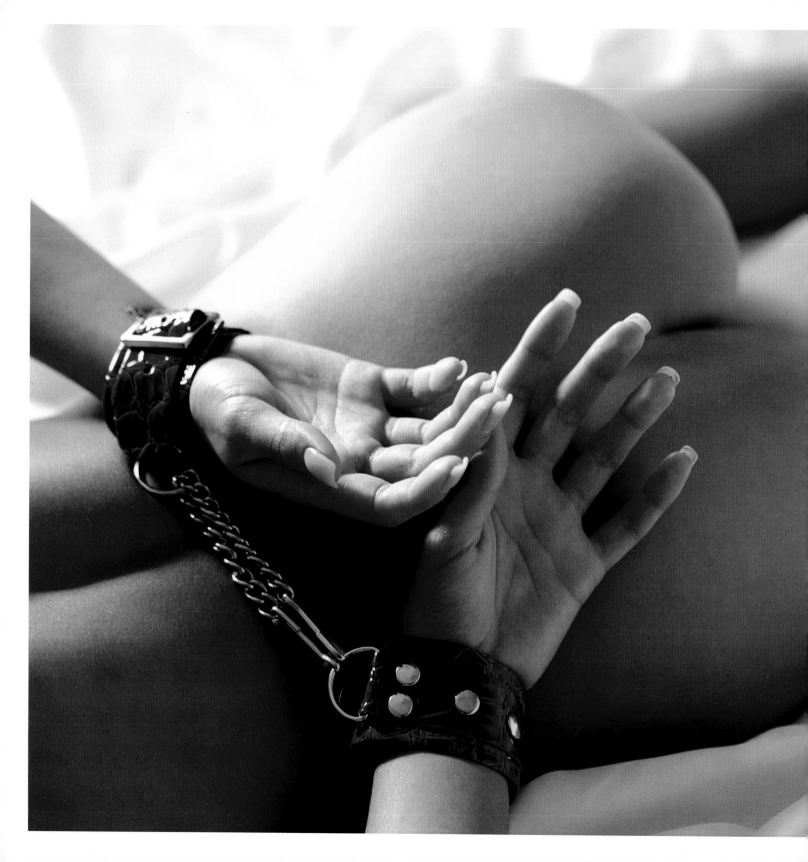

07 *Props and Toys*

Sometimes all you need to ramp up your sex life are a few sexy props. From household items like neckties and spatulas to powerful vibrators and anal beads, your options are almost limitless. But before you run up a hefty tab shopping for every toy under the sun, survey your options and play with some of the objects you already have on hand: Silk scarves can double as blindfolds, and an unused fly swatter can make for a great spanking device. Once you know what turns your crank, you can start adding to your collection to fill your bedside drawer with saucy objects of which the sight alone will excite your senses and set a sensual mood.

LUBE

Lube is fundamental to smokin' hot sex! This is because your options for stroking, pulsing, squeezing, twisting, rubbing, grinding, and kissing multiply exponentially when you're both nice and wet. Remember the Slippery Palm (page 79), the Temple (page 92), and the Twist and Shout (page 83)? Of course you do! These moves are packed full of climactic pleasure, but without lube, they simply wouldn't do the trick. In fact, without lube, they'd lead to pinching and chafing. Ouch!

But lube does more than allow you to perform Olympian feats you never thought possible. Research indicates that lube actually leads to higher levels of arousal, pleasure, and satisfaction. A study of 2,453 women found that the use of water- and silicone-based lubricants significantly decreased symptoms of sexual dysfunction, and 70 percent of participants reported that their sexual experiences were enhanced by using it.

Though some people are concerned that using lube can feel clinical or dampen the sexual mood, one experience with the slippery stuff should do the trick to convert the non-believers. Even putting it on can be hot and exciting, so experiment with different modes of application:

Put some lube in the palm of your hand and make a fist, allowing the liquid to slowly drip all over her thighs.

Rub it all over your breasts as you look into your partner's eyes and then slide your slippery boobs all over his sweet spots.

Sensually apply lube to your lips and then use your wet lips to spread it all over your partner's hot zones.

Use a soft paintbrush or makeup brush for a slow, sensuous application.

Use a flavored lube with a heavy hand and then lick off the excess goodness.

Refrigerate your favorite lube for a few hours and play with the cool tingle in your mouth while you go down on your partner. Alternate with a sip of hot water or tea to play with temperature and keep your partner guessing.

Rub your hands together and use your breath to warm the lube before stroking your partner.

Add some dirty talk to the mix: "I want my pussy even wetter so you can slide in your huge cock," or "I'm going to make my dick nice and slick so I can pound you with it."

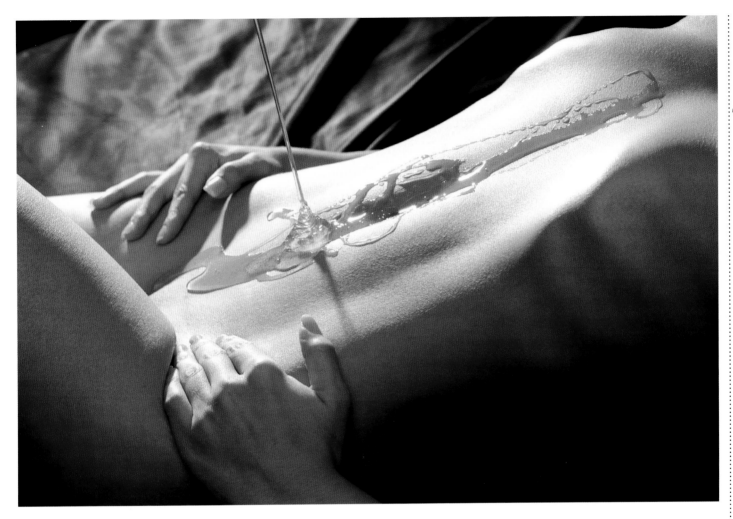

Water-based lubes are condom-safe, great for intercourse, and wash away with ease. Check out Blossom Organics, Hathor Aphrodisia, and Liquid Silk, which contain natural ingredients and have a light, neutral taste. Silicone-based lubes tend to be more slippery and longer lasting, making them ideal for anal play, hand jobs, and sex underwater. My favorites include Überlube and Pink Silicone, which both contain the moisturizer vitamin E.

A woman's lubrication does not always reflect her arousal levels. In fact, there are a variety of factors that can impact vaginal lubrication including diet, stress, medications, menstrual cycle, and hormone levels. I often hear women bragging that they get wet "like a faucet" or lamenting that they're "dry like a desert." Neither of these scenarios is necessarily grounds for celebration or grief, and there is nothing wrong with using bottled lube to enhance the experience.

REAL PEOPLE, REAL SEX

"I have a lube trick that has been good for my love life and his ego. Every night, before I go to bed, I slip into the bathroom and rub a little on my lips . . . down there. He doesn't notice every night, but when he does, he gets all excited! I was worried that all that lube might cause problems, but my doctor assured me that the daily moisturizing is actually good for me!" –Charlene, 71

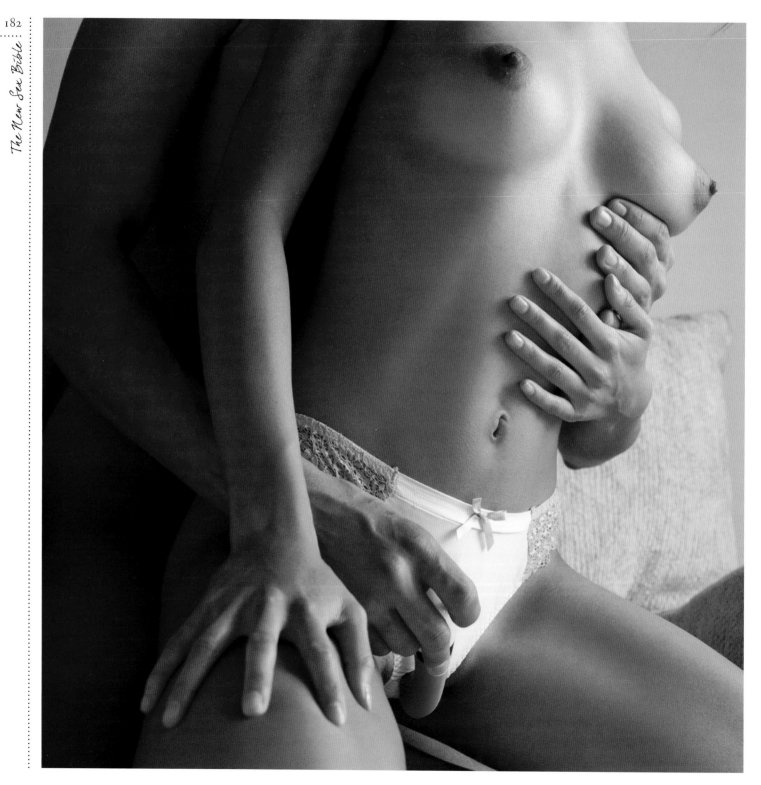

VIBRATORS

Vibrators are a common bedside prop for both men and women, and it is no surprise that their use is positively correlated with higher rates of orgasm and sexual satisfaction. Though many people assume that vibrators are universally phallic, these toys actually come in a wide range of shapes, sizes, and colors. In fact, many vibrators are designed with discretion in mind and look more like everyday items (e.g., lipstick cases) and design pieces than naughty novelties.

Vibrators can be used on various body parts including the breasts, thighs, penis, scrotum, perineum, vulva, clitoris, and vagina. Women most commonly use vibes to stimulate the clitoris (84 percent) followed by the vagina (64 percent), and men are most likely to have used toys with a lover. In fact, partnered vibrator use is so common that 94 percent of men who use vibrators report that they have done so with a partner.

Rubbing/cupping vibes are often the most effective for women, as they are perfectly shaped to cup the vulva (and by extension the clitoral complex) from top to bottom. The We-Vibe Touch allows for perfected control and rubbing, and the Spirit Leaf vibrator fits neatly between your legs for added friction.

Bullet vibes are small, often powerful vibes shaped like a large bullet or small egg. Some are attached to a remote control and others are wireless. There are also models that attach to a cock ring to provide dual stimulation during partnered sex play and those designed to be worn in conjunction with underwear beneath your clothing.

Penis-shaped vibes abound and some offer a variety of textures and modes including pulsation, rotating, and wave-like sensations. Among the most popular models are the Ellove Silicone vibrator and the Rabbit Habit Elastomer vibrator.

Super powerful vibes are perfect for those of us who just can't seem to get enough of those good vibrations! If you fall into this category, you might want to check out the classic Hitachi Magic Wand, which comes with a number of inspiring attachments, or the portable, battery-powered Mystic Wand.

Though most sex toys can be used alone or with a lover (or two!), some toys are specifically designed for couples. Try some *couple vibes*. The We-Vibe III is a C-shaped vibrator that is designed to stimulate the clitoral glans, G-spot, and penile shaft simultaneously. Controlled via remote control, it can be worn during intercourse for mutual pleasure. Some couples also wrap it around the base of his penis during the early stages of arousal until she is primed for penetration.

FAQ: THERE ARE SO MANY MODELS TO CHOOSE FROM. HOW DO I KNOW WHICH VIBRATOR IS RIGHT FOR ME?

Carlyle Jansen, sex coach and founder of Good For Her in Toronto, agrees. "The options can be overwhelming! Versatility is key for a first toy: Choose one long and thin for many internal and external possibilities. Pulses and multiple speeds also enhance pleasure options. Look for body-safe materials such as silicone or elastomer. A soft toy is best for thrusting while a firm toy is generally better for pressure and power. A powerful toy is best for those who have a hard time reaching orgasm. Look for quality toys with brand names, usually with a warranty, because they last for years and are often eco-friendly and rechargeable. In the end, because everyone is different, calling or visiting a knowledgeable sex shop is the best way to find the one best suited to you."

MAKE THE MOST OF YOUR VIBES

Not sure what to do with your vibe, now that you've got it? Aside from the obvious, give these ideas a whirl:

Wrap a bullet vibe up as a gift for your lover and ask her to wear it out in public. If it has a remote control, you can take the reins and get really creative as you get her all riled up while in line for movie tickets.

Press a powerful vibrator against your cheek while giving a blow job so that he can feel the reverberations as you suck away.

Let her work her own magic on herself with her favorite toy while you lick, kiss, slurp, breathe, suck, and twirl around it. As she takes the lead, you enhance the sensations to bring her over the edge.

Combine sensuous cock sucking with some titillating vibrations against his other orgasm hot spot—the prostate. Press a flat vibe against the patch of skin just in front of his pucker, and if he wants more, invest in a curved vibe designed specifically for prostate play. Aneros makes a number of models with his pleasure in mind.

Incorporate vibrators into your partnered sex routine. Play with them against the clitoris, anus, nipples, and perineum during intercourse.

Slide a small vibe inside of her as you devour her pussy. You can even slip your tongue in to press the vibrating toy into her hottest spots with greater pressure.

Have him sit on a flat vibrator as you go down on him so that the vibrations travel from his perineum to the inner bulb of his cock.

Let her grind her clit against a larger vibrator as you slide in from behind.

Add a vibrator into the mix right when you're about to orgasm to intensify the contractions and wave of pleasure.

COCK RINGS

Cock rings are the perfect sexual accouterment for the man who likes the feeling of a snug fit around the base of his cock. Designed to trap the blood inside of the penis, they offer the sensation of a harder, fuller erection, and though some men find that they help them to maintain a hard-on for an extended period of time, others report that the added sensation actually increases their sensitivity, resulting in an earlier onset of orgasm. Regardless of whether the ring makes you last longer or come faster, the result is usually a more intense orgasm.

There are several types of cock rings, ranging from stretchy and adjustable to textured and vibrating. Some rings sit at the base of the penis and others wrap all the way around the penis as well as the back of the testicles.

O-shaped cock rings fit around the base of the penis and can be used to help hold a condom in place. Some of them include a vibrating bullet that can be positioned against his testicles or used to rub against her clitoris during intercourse. Stretchy and adjustable rings are ideal for beginners, as the solid (non-adjustable) models can be donned and removed only when your penis is soft.

Adjustable or snap-on rings can be worn either around the penis or all the way around the base of the shaft and balls. Often made of leather or synthetic materials, these rings can be adjusted with snaps or a sliding bead.

DR. JESS SAYS . . .

Though cock rings can offer a slight increase to the size and firmness of an erection, you don't want to overdo it. If it's your first time wearing a ring, try it out for five minutes on an erect penis to make sure it fits, and be sure to remove it if you ever observe any pronounced swelling.

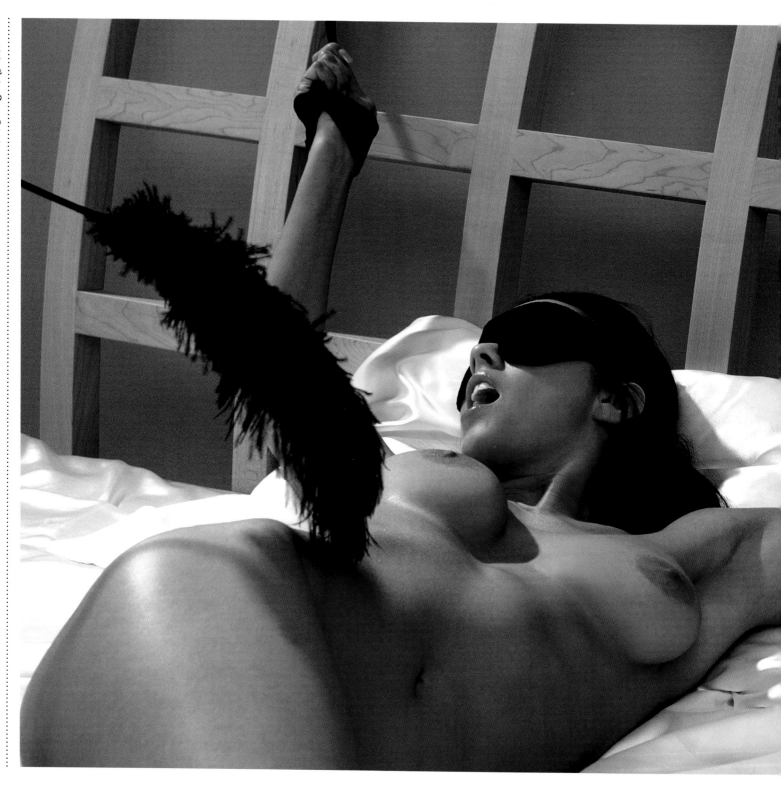

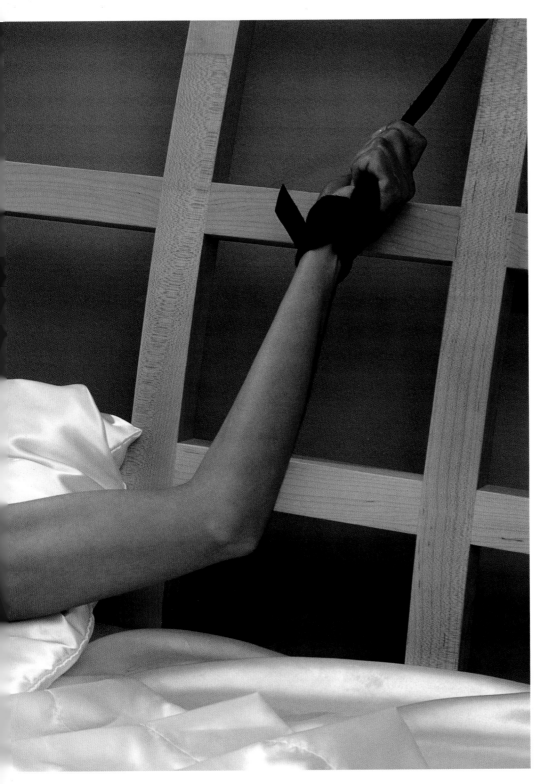

RESTRAINTS

Handcuffs, scarves, and ties take any sex act or position to new heights! Start with household items to tie your lover's hands together while you bend her over and pound her from behind, or tie him to an armchair while you drop to your knees for an unforgettable fellatio session.

Simply the sight or thought of restraints can be enough to tease your lover into a frenzy of desire, so use them to light the spark before you make it to the bedroom. Leave a pair of handcuffs on his driver's seat before he leaves for work, or place your "special tie" in her panty drawer in the morning as an indication of what you have in store for later in the evening. Who knows! She may even be inspired to greet you at the door wearing nothing but your tie . . .

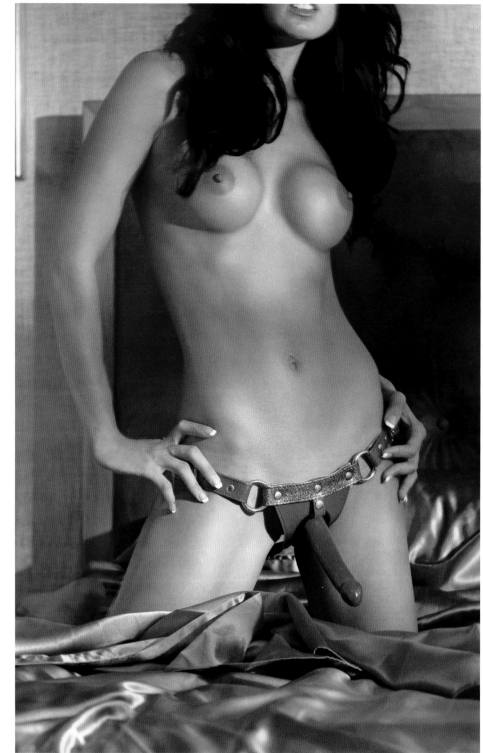

DILDOS AND STRAP-ONS

Designed to reflect the shape of a penis, dildos can be used for self-stimulation or partnered play. Some models can also be used with straps or harnesses that attach them to the body so that they can be used hands-free. Both men and women can wear and be penetrated by strap-ons. Pegging, which refers to a woman penetrating her male partner's butt while wearing a strap-on, can be a transformative experience. As couples switch roles in terms of penetration, they can learn to recognize and empathize with the emotions, sensations, and physical reactions their lover experiences during intercourse.

But dildo and strap-on use goes way beyond intercourse. Both can be used for masturbation, and strap-ons are the perfect toy for kinky sex play. You might want to press it against your lover's face as an indication of your dominance, roll it between her butt cheeks as a kinky tease, or fellate your partner's strap-on for visual effect. They're also perfect for double penetration and added stimulation during a steamy oral session.

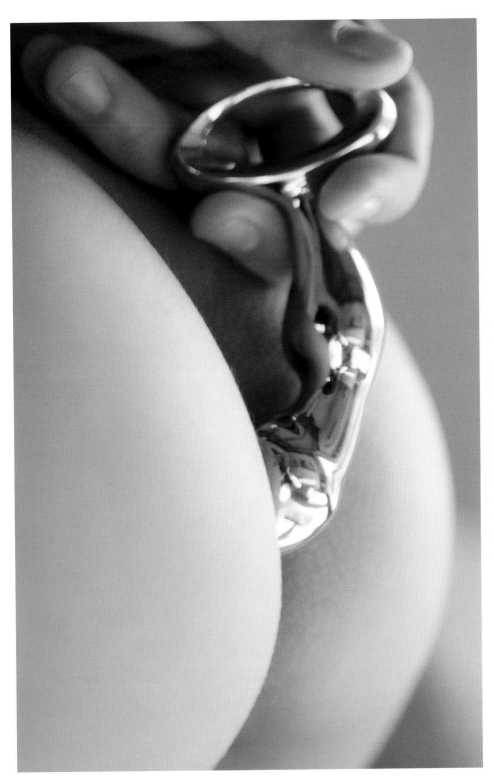

BUTT PLUGS AND ANAL BEADS

Butt plugs differ from dildos, as they have a flared base to ensure that they don't get lost in the nearly never-ending bum. They come in various shapes and sizes, and some are curved to stimulate the prostate while others vibrate for added sensation. Slide one in your lover's ass while sucking his cock or licking her pussy, or wear one yourself while on your knees taking it all in. Insertion alone might be enough to tickle your fancy, but if you want to up the ante, you can slide it in and out or twirl it around in gentle circles.

Or experiment with anal beads, which are strung together by a piece of soft rubber with a loop at the outer end for safety. Insert them one at a time and tug gently on the loop to roll them around the inside of the sensitive bum. Double your pleasure by combining them with vibrations against the clit, balls, perineum, or pucker. Removing them can be just as fun, and you may want to time popping them out one at a time with your orgasmic contractions.

KINKY PROPS

Kinking up your sex life is a great way to keep the fires burning for years to come, and there is no universal way to practice kink. Kinky sex can be rough, serious, wild, and hard-core, but it can also be playful, gentle, soft and lighthearted. If you've ever experimented with blindfolds or played with dominance and submission in the bedroom, kink is probably already on your radar. Whether you're curious about whips, gags, and riding crops or feathers, leather lingerie, and warming massage oil, kinky props offer the perfect foray into this exciting world of sensual pleasure.

BLINDFOLDS

Blindfolds are the perfect gateway prop if you want to kink up your sex life. They increase feelings of vulnerability, augment the need for trust (and submission), and force you to focus on your other senses. The sensory deprivation associated with being blindfolded takes your erotic anticipation to a new high as your lover teases, torments, kisses, tickles, or spanks you in all the right places.

GAGS

Gags range from simple cloth items you stuff in your honey's mouth to minimize sound to more advanced ball-and-strap contraptions that are higher risk due to their impact on breathing ability. Safety precautions are of paramount importance when using any type of gag, and you will need to develop a safe signal (like two finger taps or a raised hand) to indicate that you want your lover to slow down or stop.

A cloth gag involves a strip of fabric that is tied around your head so that it either covers your mouth and nose (bandit style) or fits in between your teeth to form a cleave gag.

Ring gags are made of plastic or metal and fit inside your mouth to force it agape during sex play.

Ball gags involve a small ball attached to two straps that wrap around the head. Some balls are tapered in the back for comfort and others are perforated to facilitate breathing. Never use a loose ball without straps, as this can create a choking hazard.

A stuff gag (fabric objects like underwear, bras, or stockings) is shoved into your partner's mouth. If you choose to use one, be sure to leave some material hanging out to facilitate removal.

If you want to dominate your man, shove your panties in his mouth and demand complete silence as you suck him to the heights of ecstasy. And if you want to drive her wild, use a ring gag to muffle her screams while you put your fingers, tongue, and a vibrating toy to good use between her legs.

CLAMPS

Clamps are the perfect toy for exploring the hazy pleasure/pain divide. Although you can purchase sex-specific body clamps designed for both physical sensation and aesthetic appeal, you can also use household items like bobby pins and spring-loaded paperclips (with smooth edges) as stand-ins. Try them on your nipples, labia, areolae, scrotum, or penis, proceeding gradually to test your pain thresholds. If you enjoy the sensations, you may want to invest in nipple suckers, vibrating clamps, or bell clamps that warn your lover of every movement.

Once you've discussed your boundaries with your lover, use clamps to heighten your kinky experience: Tie him up to a chair and get him all riled up. A wet hand job or blowjob should do the trick! Once he's highly aroused, apply a loose clamp to his lips and another to his nipple. His pain threshold will increase as his arousal heightens, so be sure to keep sucking and stroking away as you remind him that you run the show and are going to use his body for your pleasure alone.

WHIPS AND FLOGGERS

Excite the senses in more ways than one! The sound of a whip and the scent of hot leather can spike your arousal before these implements even make contact with your body. Throwing a single-tail whip requires instruction and practice, as it can inflict serious pain and injury, so if you want to include whipping in your sexual repertoire, check out how-to workshops and videos available at your local sex-positive store.

Floggers are composed of multiple flat tails of leather or other material attached to a short handle. They are usually shorter and softer than whips and can be applied with care over the upper back, buttocks, and chest.

KINKY OUTFITS

From leather and lace lingerie to cock harnesses and leather chaps, many kinksters find that dressing up makes the whole experience more fun and erotic. Shopping together (online or in person) helps to build anticipation, and wearing your new props and outfits sets the mood for a fully engaged encounter. If your lover has been asking you to be more assertive in the bedroom, a leather outfit may be just what you need to help you take on a more dominant role. And if you want to play the submissive, some innocent lingerie or younger clothing may help you to slip into this role more naturally and make it all the more convincing.

DR. JESS SAYS . . .

Kinky sex and BDSM (bondage, discipline, dominance, submission, sadism, and masochism) are often inaccurately represented in popular media. Kinksters are frequently depicted as mentally ill, emotionally unstable, or victimized by abuse, but research continues to confirm that these stereotypes are categorically unfounded. Being kinky is not a diagnosis, and those who enjoy kink play are no more likely to have been abused than those who prefer vanilla (non-kinky) sex. Moreover, kinky sex play is underscored by respect, consent, and care, and kinky relationships often require ongoing communication about desires, boundaries, and fears, which creates openings for a deepened connection.

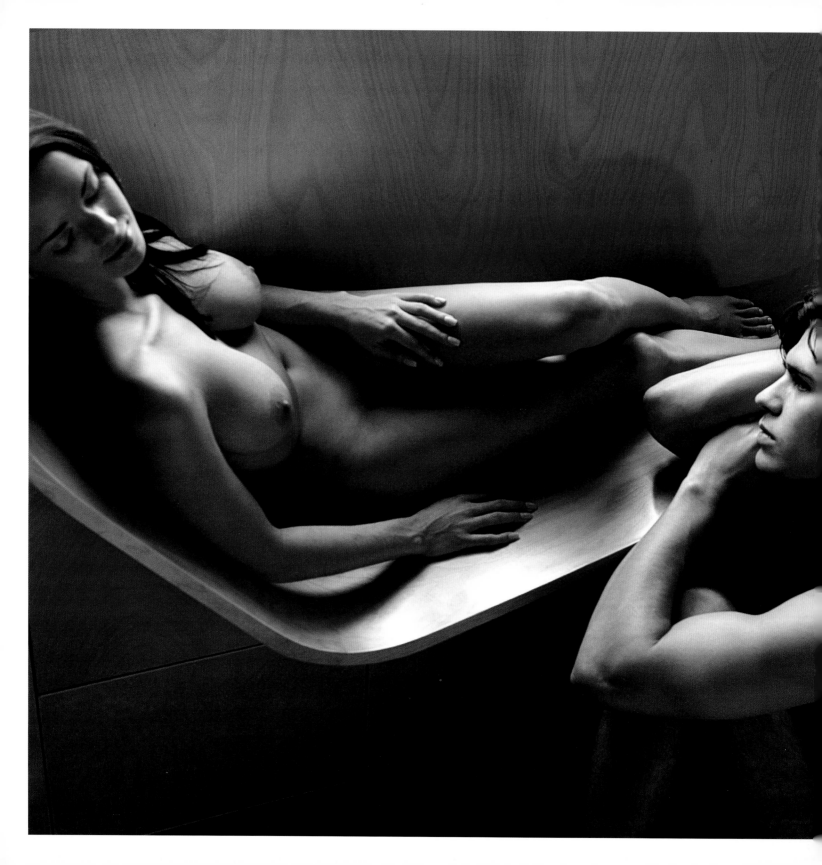

♂08 *Overcoming Sexual Challenges*

Nobody's sex life is perfect, and every single one of us runs into roadblocks at some point in time. Though strong communication skills, deep connection, comprehensive knowledge, and ongoing practice can help stave off some of the common challenges associated with desire, arousal, erection, and orgasm, problems will inevitably arise. When they do, the first step toward resolution is to take it easy on yourself and your lover. Though sex is a serious topic, a light-hearted attitude and a healthy sense of humor can help to alleviate some of the undue pressure.

LOW SEXUAL DESIRE

Levels of sexual desire fluctuate over the course of a lifetime, and ebbs and flows are perfectly normal. A decline in desire is not necessarily an indication of a problem, and there is no ideal baseline for levels of desire. If, however, *you* feel that your desire for sex is lower than your own personal ideal, consider implementing strategies to boost your interest in sex.

The causes of a decline in sexual desire are varied. Hormonal fluctuations, health issues, smoking, stress, fatigue, medications, and mental health concerns can impact our levels of desire.

Age may also play a role, as levels of desire and sexual activity tend to decrease in later years. However, there are exceptions to this rule, and though frequency of sex may decline with age, the quality tends to increase.

Some people also lose interest in sex for practical reasons. When a relationship is a source of distress, sex often tapers off, and when we struggle with poor body image, our desire can also disappear. Improving communication and levels of intimacy provides a foundation for rebuilding desire, as does engaging in activities that boost our self-esteem. Sex may also lose its appeal on account of predictability or boredom, so a more straightforward fix might involve novel experimentation.

If you have reason to believe that a decline in desire may be related to a medical issue, schedule a checkup with your medical practitioner to voice your concerns. Medical treatments may include a change in medications or hormone therapy administered via cream, patch, pill, or suppository ring. Bear in mind that these treatments do not offer a quick fix, nor do they address personal, relationship, or lifestyle issues that impede desire.

As sexual desire is a complex experience connected to many facets of your life, the process of boosting desire is highly individual. However, there are things you can do to reclaim desire over time.

Exercise is one of the most effective ways to boost sexual desire, as it can increase testosterone levels as well as augment confidence and desirability. Eighty percent of men and 60 percent of women who exercise two to three times per week feel sexier, and those who get their sweat on four to five times per week rate their sex lives as higher than average.

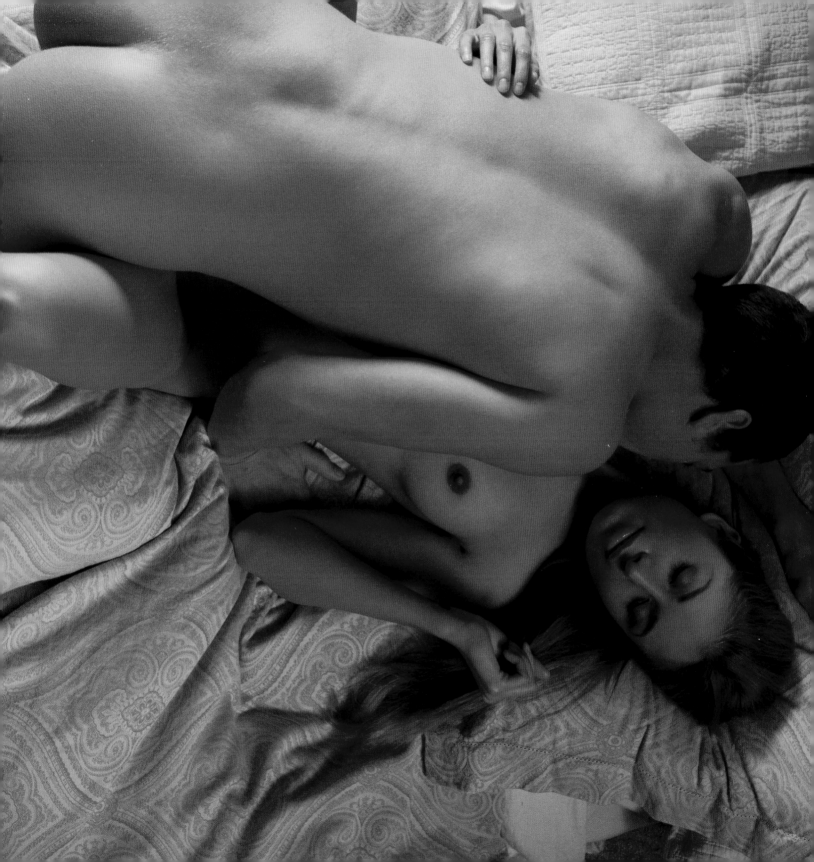

Masturbation is elemental to increasing desire in many cases, as it helps us to learn about our own bodies and reactions. Self-pleasure also increases the likelihood of orgasm and is connected with higher self-esteem. Moreover, as your body relishes in the dopamine and endorphin release, you are likely to crave more, resulting in an increase in desire for sex.

Fantasizing and engaging with erotic materials (e.g., stories, images, videos) is a fun way to learn more about your personal turn-ons and increase your desire for sex.

Kegels (page 24) can work wonders for your sex drive, as you strengthen the muscles that are responsible for sexual response and orgasm. They also improve circulation and draw awareness to your pelvic region.

Experiment with different approaches, techniques, and role-plays to discover new pathways to pleasure. Do not get hung up on the act of sex, but engage in playful games, affection, and other types of touch to reignite passion in your body and mind.

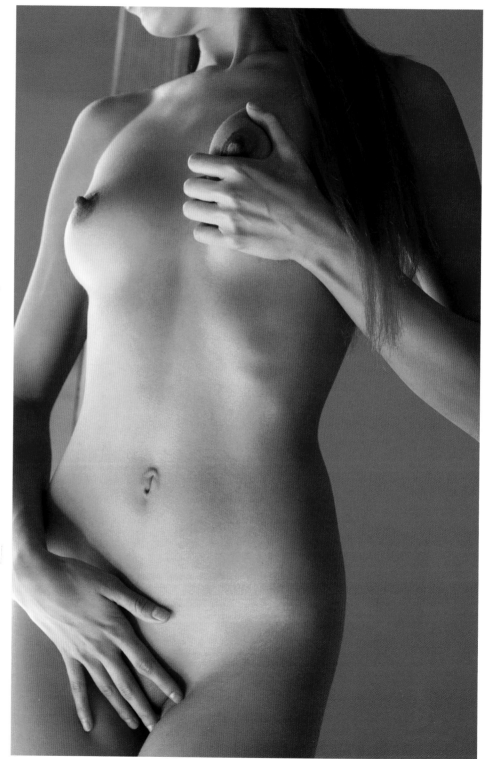

DIFFERENTIALS IN DESIRE

Every couple experiences differentials in desire at some point in their relationship, as each of our appetites for sex is as individual as our fingerprints. It would be ludicrous to attempt to eat the same meals, in the same quantity, at the exact same time as another person everyday for the rest of your life. Similarly, you cannot expect to share a perfect sex life with one person in a corresponding fashion without conflict and compromise. Even if your levels of desire are alike, they may peak at different times, and the practical elements of your individual jobs, familial responsibilities, and social interactions will inevitably create untimely differences. These disparities are not an indication of incompatibility but simply evidence that, like all good things, sexual affinity takes work.

We often assume that men want sex more than women, and developmental theories attempt to highlight this discrepancy with a link to our evolutionary past. However, the reality is that gendered generalizations often paint an inaccurate picture of desire and impede couples from resolving the challenges that arise from desire differentials. For example, the boys will be boys mentality suggesting that men are simply sex-hungry cavemen paired with the confining depiction of women as frigid victims is not only flawed but also compounds desire issues when the gender roles are reversed—which they often are.

Research not only reveals that both men and women think about sex often (approximately 18 and 9 times per day, respectively) but also that our sexual thoughts are shaped by social norms (e.g., fear of social rejection for women)—not just evolutionary imperatives. When inaccurate data, such as the myth that men think about sex every seven seconds, become a part of our cultural consciousness, it can take a toll on our sexual expression and self-esteem. Buying into pop statistics and citing them to our supposed advantage will prove futile in addressing differentials in desire. Instead, accepting that each of our sexual experiences, including desire levels, is unique and valid is essential to resolving concerns.

Acknowledging that "normal" encompasses a wide range of desire levels is the first step toward finding common ground. Desiring sex often does not make you a pervert, and desiring little or no sex does not make you a prude. The likelihood of meeting exactly at the halfway point is low, and pressuring your lover to do so will only be counterproductive. The greatest predictor of sexual compatibility is not libido but the willingness to put in a similar amount of effort to make it fulfilling.

Our levels of desire, like all of our body's needs, change with time, so ongoing communication is necessary even if your libidos seem to match up in the beginning. It can be frustrating to discover that your lover wants sex less often than you do, and it is not uncommon for the more desirous partner to feel rejected and discouraged. On the flip side, the other partner often encounters feelings of inadequacy and undue pressure. It is not uncommon for sex to cease altogether in response to this disparity, as resentment builds from both ends. What's worse is that this sexual hiatus is often accompanied by a downturn in affection, intimacy, and emotional connection.

As always, putting pressure on yourself or your sweetheart will only detract from sex, pleasure, and a happy relationship, so be gentle, offer reassurance, and make requests as opposed to complaints when talking about this sensitive subject.

REAL PEOPLE, REAL SEX

"I never thought I'd lose interest in sex, but having a child changed that. For the first time, I wanted it less often that he did, and neither of us knew how to handle the situation. I didn't even want to hug him because I was afraid it would lead to sex. This only made matters worse. One of the things that helped me to get back to my normal self was spending time alone. For the first two years of my son's life, I can't even remember being alone for more than five minutes. It's like I lost myself. As my husband started helping out more with parenting and household chores, some of the pressure was relieved and I had time to actually think about sex." –Vanessa, 35

Focusing on the quality of your sex life as opposed to the quantity of sex you have can also steer you toward greater sexual satisfaction. Getting hung up on numbers or counting the days, weeks, or months between sexual encounters can make sex seem chore-like and further intensify resentment.

If you want sex more often than your lover, take care of yourself and consider novel ways to include him in the action. Perhaps he can watch, hold you close, or lend a hand to the cause. Conversely, if you have less interest in sex but want to boost your levels of desire, self-pleasure (even if it involves non-genital touch) can help you to view your own body in more sexual terms.

Scheduling time for sex and intimacy according to a mutually agreed upon calendar can also help to address differentials in desire, particularly if the definition of sex is left open-ended. Nobody wants to be required to perform sexual activities because the clock strikes twelve, so including other acts of intimacy such as kissing, snuggling, massage, and mutual masturbation can motivate both partners to maintain the schedule.

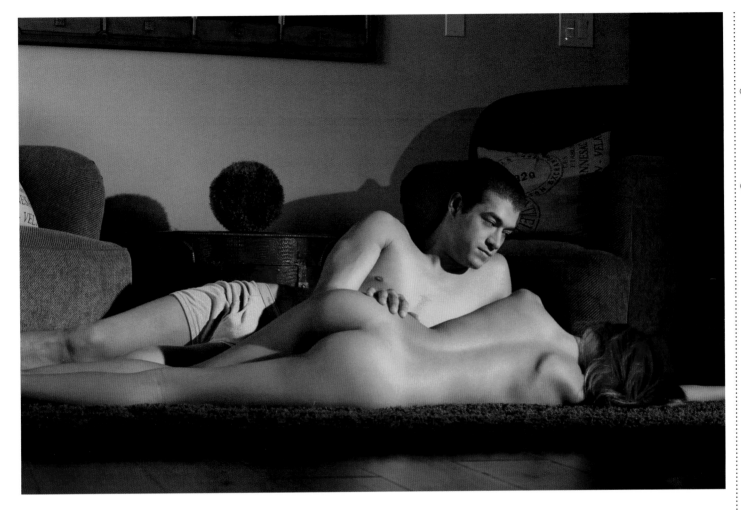

LOSS OF ERECTION

Let's face it: Our bodies don't always cooperate with us. For men whose erections disappear at an inopportune time, the stress and embarrassment can be overwhelming, but it doesn't have to be. Men may have trouble getting or maintaining an erection for a variety of reasons ranging from medical side effects to stress and anxiety. Research suggests that erectile issues may be a sign of a medical condition, so if you are experiencing repeated erection loss, check in with your doctor to rule out any medical issues.

Some of the medical conditions that can interfere with erection include pelvic surgery, spinal cord injury, heart disease, diabetes, multiple sclerosis, hardening of the arteries, Parkinson's disease, high blood pressure, as well as a number of medications. Should your erection loss be a result of one of these conditions, options for medically supervised treatment might include a change to your medications, oral prescriptions, penis pumps, injections, implants, or hormone therapy. Many men immediately seek pills in response to erectile issues, but these medications are not a solution to issues of desire, intimacy, stress-induced dysfunction, and performance pressure.

If you receive a clean bill of health from your doctor and you find that you still lose your erection, fret not! Every man will experience erection loss at some point in time, so rest assured that you are not alone. If you are in the middle of sex play when your erection disappears, don't stop what you're doing. You may have to make adjustments, change the pace, or try a new position, but keep doing what feels good for *you*. Enjoying sex play, connection, and intimate affection can boost your mood and even restore blood flow to your genital region.

REAL PEOPLE,
REAL SEX

....

"At first it was the elephant in the room. We
didn't talk about it at all and so I assumed
she was angry or embarrassed. Of course,
she assumed the same and the silence was
deafening. One day, she basically explained
that it was no big deal and asked me to go
down on her. The bells went off in my head
and I realized that we could still have sex—in
a different way. After that 'aha' moment, I
stopped putting so much pressure on myself
and my body rewarded me with more reliable
hard-ons." –Brad, 55

....

Lifestyle factors impact sexual response, so practical changes can have an impact on how your penis responds during sex play. Smoking and diabetes can restrict blood flow to the penis, as can carrying excess weight in your abdominal area. Regular exercise, a balanced diet, and a healthy dose of rest and relaxation can work wonders for your erections and sex life in general. If you are preoccupied with the stress of work, it is not uncommon for intrusive thoughts to sabotage even the hottest of sex sessions. And while you likely cannot eliminate work stress entirely, you may be able to reduce the pesky mind clutter through relaxation exercises, meditation, exercise, or yoga. If you are partnered, talk to your lover about your concerns and invite her to be a part of the solution.

Sometimes your erection can be elusive because of performance pressure. If this is the case, the solution is to reduce or remove the pressure. It may be easier said than done, but some of the deep breathing techniques described in Chapter 2 may help to get you started. Visualization techniques and fantasizing may help to get your head into the game and stay focused on the pleasure of sex as opposed to the pressure of performing. Fantasizing about another lover or sexual scenario is not an act of betrayal, and the escapism of fantasy may be just what you need to detach from the pressure of real life.

In the meantime, take advantage of the opportunity to explore other sexual options and connect with yourself and your lover in new ways. You may not believe it now, but many men say that changes in their erectile response were actually a blessing, as it forced them to be more experimental in the bedroom and start talking openly with their lovers about their sexual needs and emotions.

A NOTE FOR THE LADIES

If your lover loses his erection, rest assured that it has nothing to do with you. It's not your body, your touch, or your technique that is keeping him from getting it up. Be supportive and let him know that it's no big deal. Don't overdo it, but do tell him that it's okay and that it's perfectly normal. Because it really is! And then kindly demand that he continue to focus on your mutual pleasure, as sex doesn't begin and end with his penis. Show him how to push your buttons with his hands, lips, and tongue and show lots of appreciation.

Remember that you have probably dealt with similar issues yourself, as you can likely recall situations in which your arousal and desire were high but your body' response (e.g., lubrication and orgasm) did not reflect these levels. Share your thoughts and be sensitive to the fact that this is likely a very delicate issue.

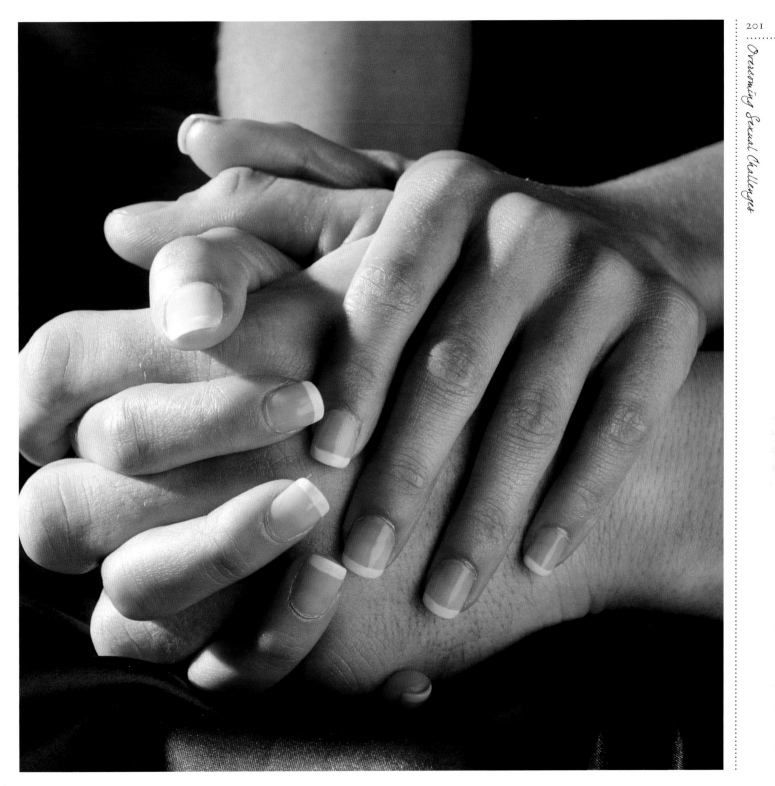

NO ORGASM

If the experience of orgasm is somewhat or entirely elusive, you are not alone. Whether you're male or female, the big Ohhh might elude you due to a lack of effective physical stimulation, intrusive thoughts, stress, or even circulation issues. But have no fear! Try these approaches to help guide your body toward orgasmic release and enjoy the journey.

Get to know your body. Oftentimes, women do not have orgasms, as we are uncomfortable or unfamiliar with our most sexual and reactive parts. As you will recall from Chapter 1, the clitoris is far more complex than most of us realize and the vulva is often integral to orgasm, yet we do not always pay it enough attention. Simply examining your genitals using a mirror can help you to learn more about this beautiful region and appreciate its splendor.

Masturbate. Most of us learn to orgasm through self-pleasure, and accepting the fact that orgasm is an experience as opposed to something a lover can "give you" can work wonders for your sexual response. Get creative during your self-love sessions and change positions, strokes, techniques, and pressure as you become acquainted with your body's reactions.

Play with toys. Women who use vibrators report higher levels of desire, arousal, and orgasm, so complement your regular routine by rolling a toy between your thighs, pressing it against your clitoral hood, or sliding it in around the opening of your vagina. Men who have difficulty reaching orgasm also benefit from the power of vibrations. Some enjoy the reverberations of a cock ring with a built-in bullet vibrator, while others prefer to rub a powerful toy against the back of the perineum to awaken the orgasmic sensations of the prostate.

Lube up! Lube is associated with significantly higher levels of pleasure and satisfaction. It also decreases your risk of tearing, discomfort, and symptoms of genital pain. And of course, it allows us to experiment with techniques that would

be impossible, painful, and even dangerous if performed under dry conditions. For example, twisting with a tight grip can make hand jobs even hotter, but without lube this sexy technique can lead to pinching and chafing—neither of which tend to result in orgasm. Ouch!

Get wet. Playing with running water over your more sensitive spots can create intense stimulation and pleasure. Haven't you noticed that your friends with detachable showerheads are always smiling?

Do your Kegels and squats. These simple exercises (page 24) encourage blood flow to the pelvic region, and circulation accelerates orgasm. The beauty of Kegels is that you can do them anywhere—in line at the grocery store, in the car sitting at a red light, riding an escalator at the mall…

Make noise. Most of us muffle or alter our sexual sounds to reflect what we hear in porn, and this can impact orgasmic tension. As we soften our groans and grunts into moans and sighs, the rhythm of our breath becomes unnatural. This breath holding impacts blood flow and oxygenation of muscles, which can impede orgasmic response. So if you feel like hollering like Tarzan, let loose and let Jane hear your primal mating call from across the jungle!

Use your body weight. Lie on your stomach and grind your body against a pillow, hand, or toy beneath your vulva. Squeeze your legs together and hump like an animal. You might feel unsexy and ridiculous at first, but your inhibitions will subside as your sexual temperature rises.

Fantasize. The brain is the engine of orgasm, so kick yours into high gear by letting your mind wander to far-off places. Whether you fantasize about being swept off your feet by a knight in shining armor or being bent over in a back alley by an aggressive stranger, allowing your thoughts to wander in pleasurable directions can increase the likelihood of experiencing orgasm.

PAIN DURING SEX

Painful intercourse, or dyspareunia, can be caused by a number of factors ranging from physical issues (e.g., infection or trauma) to psychological challenges. It affects women more often than men, with an estimated 8 percent to 20 percent experiencing persistent or recurrent pain in relation to vaginal penetration. Few studies regarding male dyspareunia have been published, but it is believed to affect between 1 percent and 5 percent of men, and symptoms may include pain in the testes, penis, or general pelvic region.

Vaginismus, which involves the sudden and painful contraction of the muscles around the vagina upon penetration, can be highly distressful. Some women find the tightening sensation so severe that they cannot handle any degree of penetration, and others describe a burning sensation that develops as penetration is prolonged or deepened. Though we don't fully understand the conditions that give rise to vaginismus, it may be linked with inflammation, injury, past trauma, vestibulodynia (hypersensitive nerve endings near the vaginal opening), stress, and psychological factors.

Because dyspareunia and vaginismus may be medically linked, talk to your doctor about your specific experiences to pinpoint or rule out medical causes. If the cause is psychogenic, you may also want to seek counseling from a professional who can support you through a program of improvement/recovery. This type of program might include exercises in breathing, relaxation, visualization, meditation, desensitization, moisturizing, Kegels, masturbation, and gradual insertions with dilators.

DR. JESS SAYS . . .

If you are looking for additional support, some physical therapists specialize in pelvic floor health. You may also want to pick up a copy of *A Woman's Guide to Overcoming Sexual Fear and Pain* by Aurelie Jones Goodwin and Marc E. Agronin.

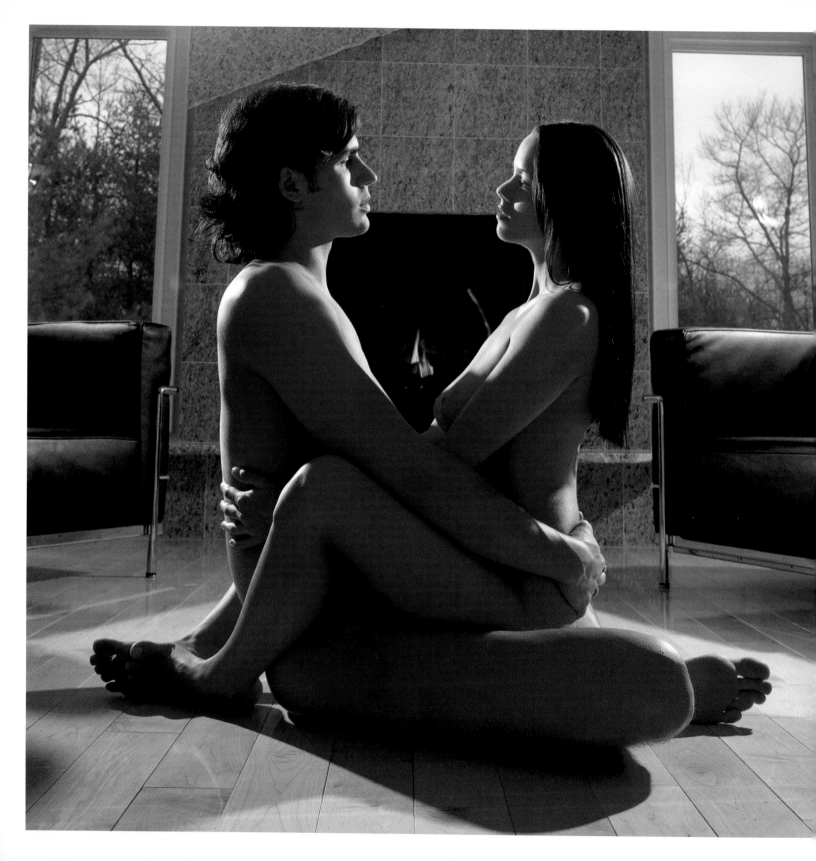

09 *Keep the Flame Burning*

If you've made it through the first eight chapters of *The New Sex Bible* you have likely accumulated the knowledge, skills, and experience to be the type of lover that everyone craves. But how do you keep the sexual flame burning as time passes? Accepting that ups and downs are a natural part of your sexual evolution is the first step toward keeping things sizzling, followed closely by the realization that it takes work to maintain a hot sex life. From practical self-help exercises to tawdry role-play suggestions, read through the following strategies designed to set your sex life ablaze for years to come.

BOOST YOUR SEXUAL SELF-ESTEEM

Confidence is sexy. And not just because experts say so! Studies reveal that confidence is one of the most sought-after traits when it comes to selecting a sexual partner. Research suggests that confident people are deemed more trustworthy and communicate more effectively. They smile, flirt, make purposeful eye contact, and speak warmly and directly. Even in photographs, women and men who appear confident are rated as more attractive by members of the opposite sex.

When it comes to sex, you have a choice between being your biggest fan or your own worst enemy. Opting for the former requires a holistic approach to cultivating self-esteem, as it is impossible to compartmentalize sexual self-confidence without considering your overall sense of self. Luckily, when it comes to sex and self-assurance, you don't have to choose between the two, as research also suggests that sex can actually boost your self-esteem.

Positive affirmations, alongside a focus on non-aesthetic components of self-esteem, have been shown to boost self-image, and the same principles can be applied to sex. By acknowledging your own strengths, sexual and otherwise, you reinforce belief in yourself, which is naturally reflected in your attitude, voice, and body language. And if you need a little help in this department, simply ask for positive feedback. While some lovers will openly sing your praises without any prompting, others will just lie back and relish in the fruits of your labor in total silence. So if you are not getting the praise you need and deserve, tell your lover to turn it up a notch! We all need positive reinforcement— especially when it comes to sex.

Learning to assert yourself is not only empowering, but asking for what you want is positively correlated with higher levels of sexual satisfaction and self-esteem. So don't be shy! Make requests, give directions, set limits, and even make demands knowing that it is good for your sex life and your sense of self.

Learning to love your body for its natural beauty is also elemental to propping up your sexual self-confidence. From exercising and eating well to positive self-talk and pampering, tap into whatever strategies work for you. And remember that it's not about gaining or losing weight, but increasing energy levels and engaging with your body in positive ways.

DEEPEN YOUR CONNECTION

When Peggy Kleinpatz and her team of sex researchers at the University of Ottawa sought to uncover sources of optimal sexuality, connection and deep erotic intimacy topped the list of components that contribute to great sex. Try these approaches to deepen your connection with your sweetheart:

Interview your lover. It doesn't matter if you've been married for thirty-three years or dating for three months. There is always something new to learn. Write down five sex- or relationship-related questions you want your lover to answer and then record your answers to one another's queries independently. When you are ready, share your answers and discuss any surprises, concerns, or points of confusion that arise. Examples of questions might include:

What was the first thing you noticed about me?

What is your favorite aspect of our sex life?

What element of our sex life would you like to improve?

What did you fantasize about the last time you masturbated?

How do you like to be touched during orgasm?

You can revisit this activity as often as you like, as both your questions and answers will evolve over time.

Be vulnerable. Authenticity has also been identified as a core component of optimal sex, and showing real vulnerability can deepen connection. As you open up to your lover, showcasing both your strengths and fragilities can be freeing and intimate.

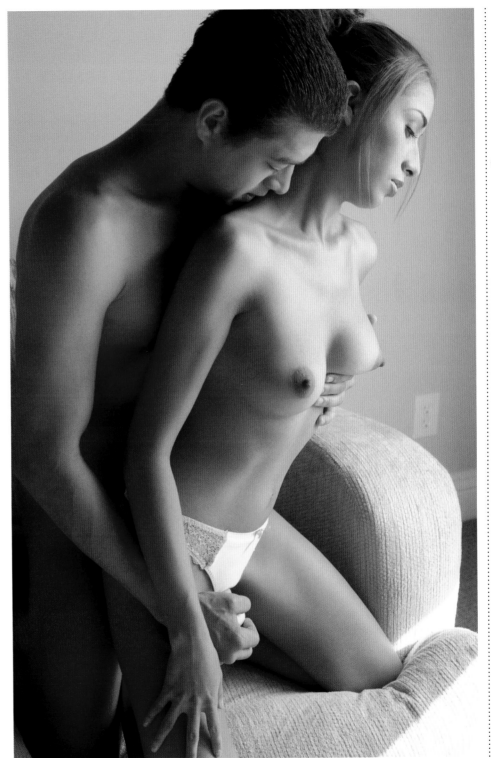

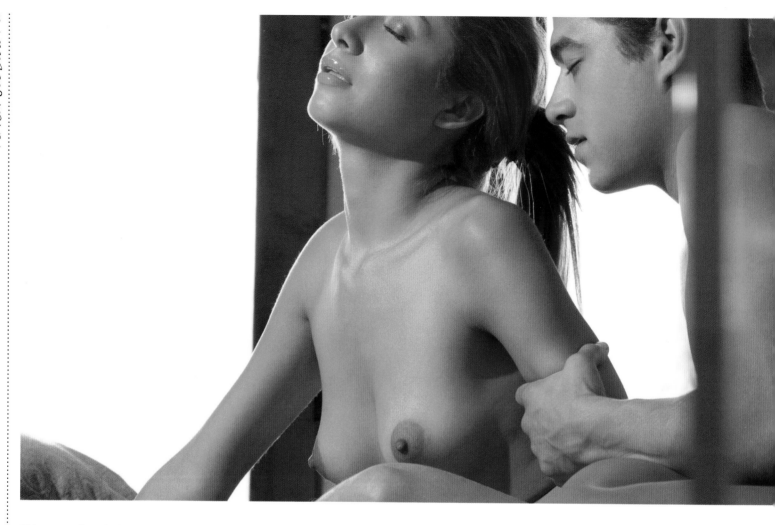

Take turns taking the lead. It is normal to fall into dominant and submissive roles in the bedroom, even if you don't refer to them as such. For example, one of you is probably more likely to initiate sex just as one of you takes control of your social calendar with greater sway. The sharing of responsibilities is healthy, but switching it up once in a while can intensify your intimate connection as you garner a deeper appreciation for the small things your lover does for you on a regular basis.

Emphasize nonsexual touch. Physical affection can deepen your bond, reduce stress, promote restful sleep, boost mood, lower blood pressure, and strengthen your immune system. Hold hands, snuggle on the couch, or just place a hand on your honey's arm when you have a conversation.

Have intense conversations. You don't need to debate the latest legislative proposal to have a heated conversation, but the open expression of feelings and desires has been shown to lead to more successful relationships. When we share parenting or household responsibilities, we

commonly get caught in a communication rut in which we narrow the topic of our conversations to reports of what we've done and what we plan to do. While these practical conversations are functional and inevitable, allowing them to replace intimate and personal discussions can take a toll on your intimate relationship as you shift from lovers to co-parents or roommates.

Offer support in various capacities. University of Iowa researchers found that newlyweds identify four areas in which they seek and provide support to their lovers: physical and emotional, esteem, informational, and tangible. As you explore new

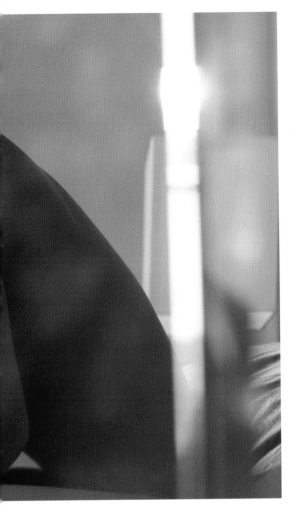

FANTASY

Sexual fantasies are common and varied, but the experience of engaging in sexual thoughts is universal. Some people fantasize about being dominated or having threesomes, and others dream of breaking the law or getting caught in the act. Fantasies may range from fleeting thoughts to elaborate and repetitive daydreams, and for the most part, we remain satisfied with fantasies as distinct from reality. That is, we indulge in fantasies for pleasure without the need or desire to live them out in real life.

Psychologist Bruce Ellis, Ph.D., and anthropologist Donald Symons, Ph.D., are leading researchers in the field of evolutionary psychology. Their findings reveal that fantasies differ between men and women. They classify men's fantasies as more lustful, noting that men think about a greater number of partners and value visual images as more important than the fantasy of touch. Women are more likely to fantasize about the response of their lover and the themes tend to be more personal and emotional. Women also tend to focus on seduction, and the content of their fantasies builds toward explicit sexual activity more slowly.

It is perfectly normal to fantasize about people other than the love of your life, and we often switch between lovers in our dreams and fantasies. One study out of the University of Vermont revealed that 98 percent of men and 80 percent of women have fantasized about someone other than their current partner in the past two months. They also found that these fantasies increase as the relationship progresses.

Sharing your deepest fantasies with your lover can intensify your connection, and many people report that the mere act of talking about a fantasy can be highly arousing. Obviously, you need to use discretion when sharing sensitive information with a loved one, and if you are nervous about divulging your most titillating fantasies to your partner, begin with your tamer thoughts to test the waters. You may also want to frame your fantasy as part of a dream you had or something you read about in a book or magazine. Always reassure your partner that your relationship takes precedence over any sexual fantasy.

If you have difficulty tapping into your fantasies, you may want to read erotic fiction or ask your lover to share her fantasies for inspiration. There is no reason to feel guilty about fantasizing. Your fantastical desires are actually good for your sex life and can improve your relationship as you learn more about yourself and your lover. Sexual thoughts also prime your sexual response by engaging your mind with your body's desires and offer you an outlet in which you control the entire sexual situation. As you engage in fantasy, you'll likely see an increase in desire and subjective (mind-based) sexual response.

ways to support your honey, consider each of these approaches, which might include affection, compliments, gentle advice, and practical favors. Communicate openly with regard to how much and what type of support you desire and listen actively to their needs and boundaries.

Holding hands can reduce stress-related activity in your brain's hypothalamus and reduce pain. Psychologist James Coan's study of women's brain activity in response to the stress of a mild shock revealed that anxiety can be soothed by hand-holding—even a stranger's hand.

FAQ: HOW CAN I ENCOURAGE MY VERY SHY GIRLFRIEND TO TALK ABOUT HER FANTASIES? AND HOW CAN I REASSURE HER THAT MY FANTASY OF HAVING A THREESOME IS JUST A HARMLESS THOUGHT THAT TURNS ME ON? I DON'T ACTUALLY WANT TO DO IT.

Dr. Ruthie offers these words of wisdom: "I find that shy people have some of the very best fantasies. It's harder to find out what they are, but absolutely worth the loving effort. One of my favorite ways is to turn it into a sexy game. Pick out a compilation of short erotica stories together that are written with women or couples or mind, or a how-to guide like this one! Each of you can take a different colored pen and privately mark the sections, words, or ideas that sound exciting, then swap. Allow her to do it first, so she doesn't feel pressured by the things you've marked. Then, when you're done, see where your fantasies overlap and giggle about them together. Once the conversation around fantasies has been opened it may be easier to talk about how threesomes is just another one of yours, and does not reflect anything negative about the relationship or your desire for her. The two of you may even discover that she has fantasies about other partners, too!"

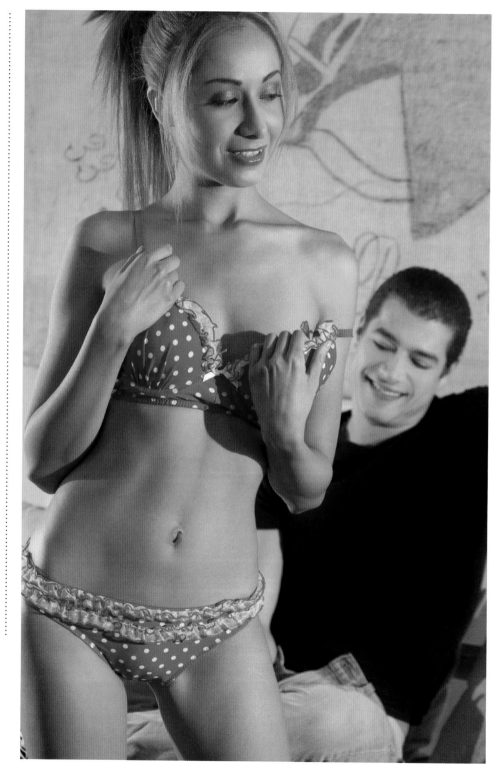

ROLE-PLAY

Engaging in role-play is the antidote to sexual monotony. During the first six to twelve months of courtship, passionate love provides enough sexual kindling to keep the flames burning, but as that period of limerence (overwhelming sense of attraction) subsides, companionate love takes over. During this equally meaningful and fulfilling stage of our relationship, we often have to cultivate desire using creative approaches. Role-playing offers the perfect solution to fuel the fire and ensure that your companionate love is accompanied by passionate love-making.

Role-plays can take on many forms and they may reflect values and desires that are entirely oppositional to those you pride yourself on in real life. Oftentimes, the most appealing roles are those that stray most significantly from our lived reality. If you manage great responsibility at work or in the home, you may derive great pleasure from indulging in a submissive role. And if you spend most of your days catering to everyone else's needs, playing a selfish role may be the perfect escape from reality. Whatever parts you decide to play, discuss them with your sweetheart ahead of time to negotiate boundaries and offer reassurance as needed.

It is not uncommon to feel self-conscious or even silly when you first try to take on a role, but turning the lights down low and waiting until you're highly aroused before slipping into character can help to temper your inhibitions. Dressing the part and assuming a fake name may also help ease you into it. As you engage more intensely with your role, it will start to feel more natural and you can stay focused on your pleasure as opposed to remaining in character.

Whether you opt to have a one-night stand with a total stranger, plan a tryst with a long-lost love, or hook up with a young lover to show him the ropes, the possibilities for role-plays are endless. Some common roles involve escorts, athletes, cheerleaders, cops, teachers, doctors, tradespeople, strippers, and dominatrixes. Scenarios might involve love affairs, casual hook-ups, threesomes, hitchhiking, rewards or punishment, blackmail, photo shoots, travel, humiliation, teasing, or dominance and submission.

TIPS FOR HOT ROLE-PLAYS

Before you embark on role-play, establish a safe word or signal that you can use if you feel uncomfortable at any point in time. This safety precaution signals to your lover that he or she should stop right away and check in to ensure your well-being.

Decide ahead of time how far you are willing to go and set clear boundaries. If there are words, scenarios, or phrases with which you are uncomfortable, steer clear of them.

Practice your dirty talk skills (see Chapter 3), as language is elemental to role-play.

Be yourself! Injecting your own personality into your new role will help ease you into character.

Base your role-play scenarios on your fantasies, changing details to ensure that you do not incite your lover's insecurities.

Don't get hung up on mainstream ideas. The pizza delivery guy and French maid can make for hot routines, but push your limits and engage in your real fantasies. Perhaps you want to be Tarzan and Jane or play out a rape scene. Just be sure to talk about your needs and boundaries ahead of time.

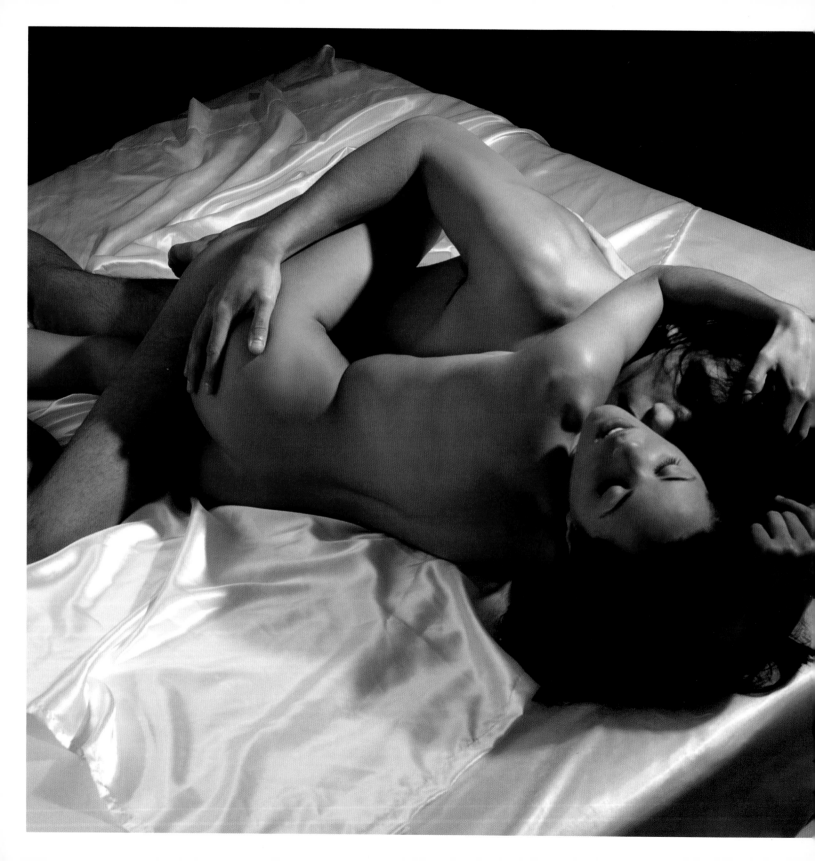

Afterword: The Happy Ending

Now that you've worked your way to the very end of *The New Sex Bible* (hopefully with a few sexual stops along the way), you probably feel quite well-versed in both the art and science of sexual pleasure. But your journey has just begun! Sex is as much a process as an experience, and in both respects it is constantly evolving. Even after you've mastered the most advanced moves and positions, you'll continue to discover new permutations that elevate your orgasms to new heights. And as you cultivate a deep connection with your lover and build your sexual self-esteem, you'll observe fluctuations in these levels over time. This, of course, is all a part of the process that makes sex exciting, appealing, and fulfilling.

I encourage you to revisit some of the content of *The New Sex Bible* from time to time to help map your own sexual journey and uncover new interpretations of pleasure. What comes easily to you today may take more effort in the future, and you're likely to find that your reactions to different techniques and positions change with time. Embracing these changes not only improves the quality of your sex life but also enriches your sexual journey by heightening the authenticity of every experience.

Once again, I'd like to express to you my deep appreciation for including me in this journey and I wish you a lifetime of happy beginnings, middles, and endings!

Resources

THERAPISTS AND COUNSELORS

The American Association of Sexuality Educators, Counselors and Therapists (AASECT)
> Maintains a global directory of certified member professionals.
> www.aasect.org/referral-directory

ONLINE SEXUALITY RESOURCES

Scarleteen.com
> Though designed for teens, Scarleteen offers some of the most comprehensive sex education and resources that can be found online, and the bulk of their content is relevant for adults, too.

GoAskAlice.com
> This site offers advice and resources on a range of sexual health topics.

PlannedParenthood.org
> Counseling for STDs, pregnancy, and other sexual health issues via online chat, telephone inquiries, and local in-person appointments.

ONLINE STORES

ThePleasureChest.com

GoodForHer.com

OhhhCanada.ca

GoodVibes.com

Babeland.com

SexyPartyWear.com

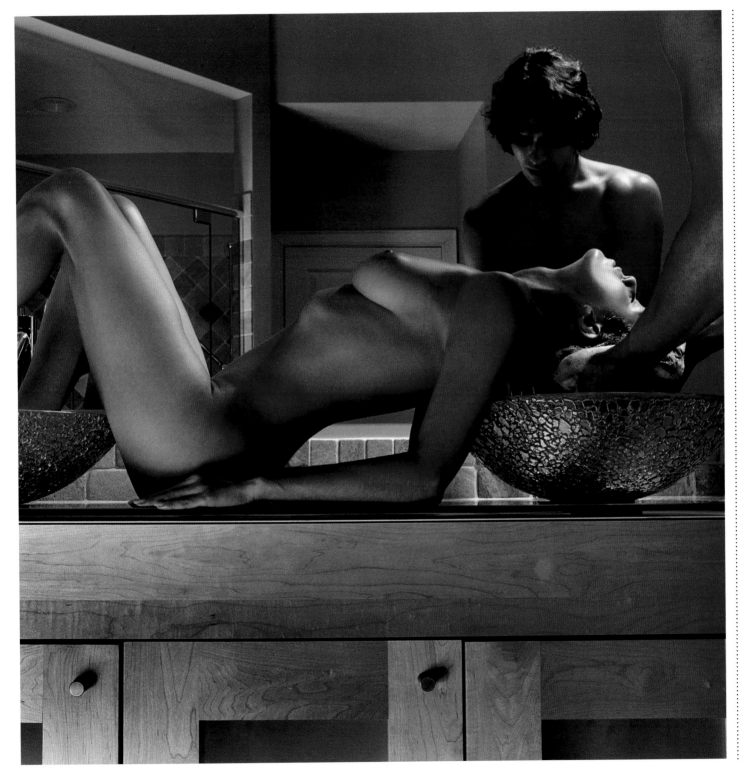

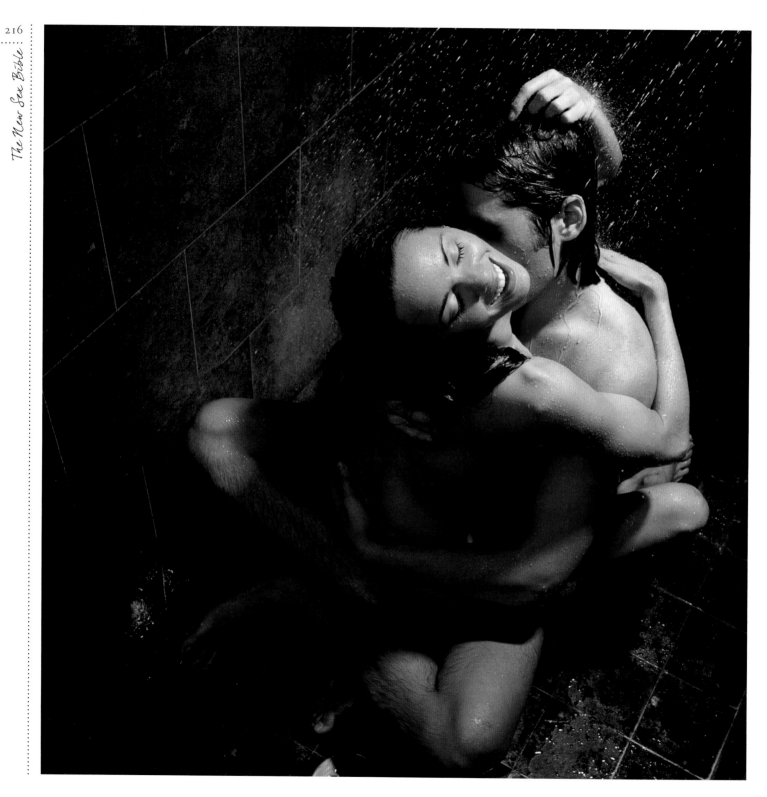

BOOKS

Mating in Captivity: Unlocking Erotic Intelligence by Esther Perel
　　Offers descriptions and case studies to explore erotic intelligence and the complexities of sustaining desire.

The Guide to Getting it On by Paul Joannides
　　A comprehensive sexuality manual that covers almost every sex-related topic imaginable.

Hot Mama: The Ultimate Guide to Staying Sexy Throughout Your Pregnancy and the Months Beyond by Lou Paget
　　A sexual handbook book for mothers to-be and new moms

The Orgasm Answer Guide
by Barry Komisariuk, Beverly Whipple, Sara Nasserzadeh, and Carlos Beyer-Flores
　　Offers straightforward answers to address every aspect of orgasm

The Ultimate Guide to Prostate Pleasure
by Charlie Glickman and Aislinn Emirzian
　　Provides an in-depth exploration of prostate play

BOOKS (KINK)

How to be Kinky by Lord Morpheous

The Little Book of Kink by Jessica O'Reilly
　　I'm shamelessly plugging my own book, because it's a great little guide with practical positions, suggestions, and techniques for newbies.

OTHER SEXUALITY-RELATED BRANDS AND SERVICES

Love Cloud
　　www.lovecloudvegas.com
　　If you want to join the mile-high club and enjoy some private time in the air, Love Cloud has you covered!

Desire Resort & Spa (Puerto Morelos, Mexico)
　　www.desireresorts.com
　　An upscale couples-only resort designed with pleasure in mind.

Hedonism II (Negril, Jamaica)
　　www.hedonism.com
　　Nude vacations for singles, couples, and groups in sunny Jamaica!

Acknowledgements

I am so incredibly grateful to work in a field as exciting, interesting, glamorous, and challenging as sexology. I know how privileged I am to have carved out a career of passion and I have so many people to thank.

To all those who opened up to share their personal stories and ask meaningful, honest questions, I offer my sincere gratitude and deep respect. Your real-life experience continues to serve as an invaluable learning tool without which this project would be incomplete.

To the brilliant experts and fellow authors who shared their knowledge and hustled to meet my tight deadlines, I am profoundly thankful and hope that I can return the favor someday soon.

To the supportive and kind team at Quiver Books, who make each of these projects a pleasure to work on, I extend my heartfelt appreciation. It truly is amazing to watch a book come to life and I obviously could not have done it

without the entire team, including Jill Alexander, John Gettings, Jennifer Kushnier, Burge Agency, Ed Fox, Regina Grenier, Leah Jenness, and Amy Paradysz. Special thanks goes to Jackson Byrne for his patience, thorough research, and thoughtful input, which were elemental to the completion of the original manuscript.

To my readers, followers, Tweeps and numerous supporters whom I've never met in-person, I thank you for the ongoing support and well-wishes. People often ask how I handle the negative pushback and resistance in a field as controversial as sexology and I respond with a reminder that the encouragement actually outweighs the resistance. Your support keeps me motivated and inspired.

Finally, to my loving partner, Brandon, thank you for being consistently awesome. Happiness is love and I'm blissfully happy.

XOXO

About the Author

Jessica O'Reilly (Dr. Jess) is a leading sex and relationship expert who loves her job just as much as she loves wine, cheese, crab, hiking, and airplane turbulence — seriously. From hosting PlayboyTV's hit reality series, *SWING,* to facilitating couples' retreats in the sunny Caribbean and the European countryside, every day is an absolute pleasure.

Dr. Jess has worked directly with thousands of singles and couples and her advice reaches tens of millions across the globe. She is regularly featured by *Cosmopolitan, Men's Fitness,*

Women's Health, The Huffington Post, City TV, Canada AM, CBC, ABC Spark, Playboy Radio, and Breakfast Television to name a few. She also engages hundreds of live audiences each year at a range of events including clinical conferences, professional development workshops, trade shows, fundraisers, community service groups, colleges/universities, and corporate retreats.

Catch up with Dr. Jess on Twitter, Facebook & Instagram by following @SexWithDrJess or check out her work online at SexWithDrJess.com.

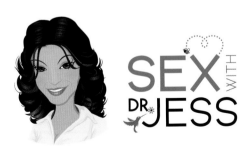

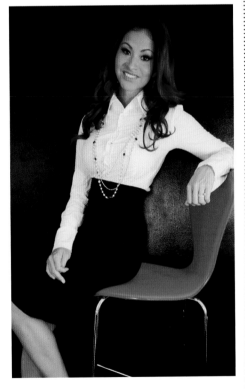

Index